ALSO BY PETER KAMINSKY

Pig Perfect: Encounters with Remarkable Swine and Some Great Ways to Cook Them

The Moon Pulled Up an Acre of Bass: A Flyrodder's Odyssey at Montauk Point

Seven Fires: Grilling the Argentine Way (with Francis Mallmann)

The Elements of Taste (with Gray Kunz)

Celebrate! (with Sheila Lukins)

John Madden's Ultimate Tailgating (with John Madden)

Happy in the Kitchen (with Michel Richard)

The Maccioni Family Cookbook (with Egi Maccioni)

Cucina of Le Marche (with Fabio Trabocchi)

Charred and Scruffed (with Adam Perry Lang)

Letters to a Young Chef (with Daniel Boulud)

American Waters: Fly-Fishing Journeys of a Native Son

The Flyfisherman's Guide to the Meaning of Life

Culinary Intelligence

Culinary Intelligence

The Art of Eating Healthy (and Really Well)

Peter Kaminsky

ALFRED A. KNOPF NEW YORK 2012

THIS IS A BORZOI BOOK
PUBLISHED BY ALFRED A. KNOPF

www.aaknopf.com

Knopf, Borzoi Books, and the colophon are registered trademarks of Random House, Inc.

Grateful acknowledgment is made to Artisan, a division of Workman Publishing Co., Inc. New York, for permission to adapt the recipe for "Roast Chicken" from *Bouchon* by Thomas Keller, copyright © 2004 by Thomas Keller; to adapt the recipe for "Double Cut Ribeye" from *Happy in the Kitchen* by Michel Richard, copyright © 2006 by Michel Richard; to reprint the recipe for "Chimichurri" from *Seven Fires* by Francis Mallmann, copyright © 2009 by Francis Mallmann; and to reprint the recipe for "Shaved Raw Brussels Sprouts with Castelrosso Cheese" from *The Frankies Spuntino Kitchen Companion & Cooking Manual* by Frank Falcinelli, Frank Castronova, and Peter Meehan, copyright © 2010 by Frank Falcinelli, Frank Castronova, and Peter Meehan. All rights reserved.

Library of Congress Cataloging-in-Publication Data
Kaminsky, Peter.
Culinary intelligence: the art of eating healthy (and really well) / Peter Kaminsky—1st ed.
p. cm.
Summary: "A formerly overweight food writer tells us how to maximize flavor per calorie so we can keep our waistlines slim without sacrificing the joy of good food"—Provided by publisher.
ISBN 978-0-307-59337-5 (hardback)
1. Cooking.
2. Nutrition.
I. Title.

TX652.7.K36 2012
641.5—dc23 2011035142
Jacket photograph by Victoria Pearson
Jacket design by Abby Weintraub

Manufactured in the United States of America
First Edition

Dedicated to Melinda

On the trip home the sun came out. Steam rose from the blacktop, bound to reassemble itself as yet another rain cloud. We stopped at a roadside watermelon stand and were greeted by the smell of fresh sawdust and the sight of sweet Navasota stripers iced down and ready to be served by the slice.

—RODNEY CROWELL,
Chinaberry Sidewalks

Contents

Culinary Intelligence

CHAPTER 1 My Occupational Hazard

Some people are born with perfect pitch. I'm not one of them, but I have something akin to that when it comes to food. I was born with a taste in my mouth, in much the same way that a songwriter is born with a tune in his head. Taste and its kissing cousin, aroma, affect me powerfully. When my downstairs neighbor browns onions, the sweet and sharp scents rise up through the stairwell of our Brooklyn brownstone, carrying with them memories of my grandmother's brisket, my mother's smothered chicken, or a street vendor's sausage sandwiches at the Feast of San Gennaro.

In the DNA lottery, I inherited a very acute palate and an equally sensitive sniffer. Just a pinch of tarragon hits me like the blast of a steam room. A couple of drops of sesame oil focuses my attention the way the scent of a trembling pheasant agitates a bird dog. I'm not saying that I can tell you what kind of oak dropped the acorns that fed the pig who ended up on my plate as a slice of Spanish ham. But I could never confuse the flesh of such a noble hog with the bland waterlogged ham from a factory-raised pig.

This obsession with taste can be a little maddening to friends and family, especially when we go to a restaurant. If, for example, a waiter passes by with a plate of coq au vin, my head will snap around as I breathe in the seductive smells. At such times I'll check out of the conversation, trying to determine exactly which herbs and spices are in a dish. It's not that I need to be right. It's a compulsive culinary crossword puzzle that I conduct with myself. I can't help it.

This isn't bragging. I'm stating a fact about myself that I only fully recognized when I was well into adulthood. Until then, I thought everyone was like me: assaulted all day long by fusillades of flavor and irresistible aromas. It took me a long time to realize that not everyone inhaled and ingested their way through life this way. In fact, only about 4 percent of the population has this, er, gift—and it explains why so many of us turn out to be chefs, restaurateurs, sommeliers, winemakers, restaurant critics, cookbook authors, and bloggers of the alliance of press and pantry that I call the "foodoisie." In a way, it's their destiny for the same reason that tall men with impressive leaping skills become basketball players, smaller men with great eye-hand coordination become golfers, socially awkward undergrads become Internet billionaires. For those of us who end up in the food world, to borrow a phrase from nouvelle-cuisine master Alain Senderens, "the table beckons." Always.

For the first half of my life, I was not fully aware that I was a member of the foodoisie. True, I loved food—eating it and cooking it—but it was a hobby, not an occupational hazard. When writing about food became my occupation, the professional pursuit of pleasure put on pounds and screwed up my body chemistry. The choice was clear: mend my munching or fast-forward to Judgment Day. In terms of a healthy diet, I realized that although I ate wonderful rarefied food I was still a typical American in my eating habits, because, whether you are scarfing down scoops of Cherry Garcia with butterscotch sauce or dining on béarnaise-bathed filet mignon and butter-browned potatoes Anna, it all puts you on a glide path to obesity, heart disease, diabetes, and all other so-called diseases of civilization. Maybe better to call them "illnesses of indulgence."

This book is the result of my truly insatiable appetite for the pleasures of the table and my equally strong urge to survive. Rather than forgo health on the one hand, or hedonism on the other, I believe that the two can coexist quite happily.

The event that brought me into the full-time food world occurred on December 18, 1994. Two days before, my daughter Lucy and I caught a dozen blackfish off Coney Island. Before then, my résumé was as typically wide-ranging and inconsistent as any freelancer's. I had been an itinerant humor writer, shuttling between magazines such as *National Lampoon* (where I was managing editor) and the life of a joke writer and producer of comedy television. It was a wacko, nerve-racking way to make a living, raise a family, and, on the first of most months, pay the mortgage. To balance out this unsettled existence, a generous act of fate guided me to the serene pastime of fishing. It took over my life, converted me into a hunting-and-fishing journalist, and eventually led to my own "Outdoors" column in the *New York Times.*

In 1994, I wrote a series of columns called "A Season on the Harbor." Each month I reported on a different fishing excursion in New York City waters. It may come as a surprise to some, but the Big Apple has 578 miles of coastline once you stretch out all the curves and crannies. It is home at different times of the year to hundreds of millions of striped bass, bluefish, shad, weakfish, lobsters, oysters, clams, and mussels. Researching those columns was heaven to me: casting into acres of striped bass beating the waves to a froth off Runway 9 at JFK (where jets with lowered landing gears came haircut close), or laying my rod across the gunwales of my boat to take in a fireworks display over the Statue of Liberty with no other soul in sight.

In early December, for the last piece in the series, Lucy and I went out for blackfish, a local quarry that looks like a mahimahi that has been mugged and left for dead. Looks notwithstanding, it is quite delicious. On a blustery but fishable day, we boarded a local pay-to-fish boat out of Sheepshead Bay, Brooklyn. The regulars huddled inside the cabin, stowing their rods in the corner and settling into the more consequential business of penny-a-point pinochle. On deck, next to Lucy and me, an affable angler named Eddie Dols pulled in fish after fish. Eddie was generous with his knowledge and showed us how to detect a bite. He had spent his working years as the keeper of Olaf, the walrus at the Coney Island Aquarium. Lucy and I left the boat with two dozen blackfish fillets in our cooler.

The next day, I had scheduled my annual Christmas lunch with my college roommate, Vinnie Farrell, at '21' Club in Manhattan. The chef was Michael Lomonaco, who has since gone on to numerous television appearances and is in the history books as the guy who went to pick up his eyeglasses rather than taking the elevator to his restaurant in the World Trade Center on the morning of September 11, 2001. I knew Lomonaco as a fellow fisherman, with whom I had shared advice on tackle, lures, and general fishing lore.

I phoned him with a request.

"Hey, Mike, I caught a bunch of blackfish. If I bring them in, could you cook some for me and Vinnie? You can sell the rest."

"No problem," he answered, as I knew he would.

The next day found me waiting in the coat-check line at '21' Club, with my little red Igloo cooler in hand and Frank Gifford and Ethel Kennedy just ahead of me. All in all, the ritziest coat-check line I'd ever been on.

"Did you bring your lunch?" Gifford asked in jest.

"As a matter of fact, I did." With that we fell into conversation. I learned that Gifford had taken the occasional striper off Long Island Sound, near his Connecticut home.

Lomonaco invited me into the kitchen. This took place before images of the controlled chaos of restaurant kitchens had become a staple of television programming. True, I had flipped burgers in summer camp in the Poconos, and worked as a counterman at Cohen's Famous Knishes in West Orange, New Jersey, but it was not until that day at '21' that I got my first glimpse of a world-class restaurant kitchen firing on all cylinders.

Like other kitchens I would get to know in the coming years, Lomonaco's moved at Mach 2: everyone shouting over each other yet somehow communicating, pans clanging, meat sizzling, the door to the dining room swinging in and out as hot plates left the kitchen and trays of empties returned. It was a symphony of aromas barely registering before they were replaced by new sensations: the perfume of rosemary on veal chops, wine clouds billowing off a superheated pan, the sizzle of burning sugar, the crackle of crisping meat, the scent of salmon so fresh it smelled like a sea breeze, and—since this was '21' Club, where money was no object (or maybe the *only* object)—healthy helpings of the season's last white truffles.

Because we were friends, Mike liberated a few shavings of

those costly beauties for an extra course of bay scallops to go along with the blackfish, which he dredged in seasoned corn-meal crumbs and sautéed in clarified butter. He served the fillets atop a bed of black olives, sun-dried tomatoes, sautéed fennel, and a sprig of fresh dill. The confluence of the holiday season, the setting, and the fact that my daughter and I had caught the main course combined for the most wonderful blackfish that anyone could ever hope to eat.

After that sublime meal, the story basically wrote itself. My editor at the *Times*, Susan Adams, liked the piece so much that she prevailed on her boss to give my story most of a page, which was unusual for the "Outdoors" column. They even ran two pictures with it: Eddie Dols reeling in a fish, and Lomonaco flipping pans in his chef's whites.

I received more letters on that one piece than all the letters combined for everything else I have ever written, with the exception of a column I wrote about 9/11. Something in this lucky turn of events spoke to me loud and clear: I needed to let my inner food guy out and find him a writing job.

Then, obeying E. B. White's maxim that people in New York must "be prepared to be lucky," I got lucky when the woman writing the "Underground Gourmet" column at *New York* magazine decided to put down her pen. My friend Kurt Andersen was *New York*'s editor in chief at the time. Earlier in 1994, I had already written my first major food article, a cover story for *New York* about the opening of Gramercy Tavern. It was a "making of" piece, all about the process of the creation of a restaurant, not the creation of meals, not really a dining piece. Still, it made a big splash and put me at the threshold of the food world. "Would you like to write 'Underground Gourmet'?" Kurt asked.

Different from the main restaurant-review column, "Underground Gourmet" celebrated the ethnic diversity of the New York foodscape as well as up-and-coming and affordable fine dining. Whereas the chief restaurant critic's job was split between piling on the plaudits for deserving restaurants and warning the public away from disappointments, the Underground Gourmet's task was to turn people on to little-known and out-of-the-way places that served great food. You either wrote a good review or wrote none at all.

I took the gig. At that time I carried 172 pounds on my five-foot-nine frame. My Levi's had a thirty-four-inch waistband, just about right for my demographic.

It was the perfect food job for me, much more in line with my tastes than writing reviews of pricey restaurants. During the years that my fishing-and-hunting writing took me into small-town America, I had made a habit of tracking down authentic heartland food, by which I mean the kind of fried, smoked, and barbecued fare traditionally consumed beyond the Lincoln Tunnel. I made a practice of including a paragraph about a restaurant here, or a recipe there, in every story I wrote.

This is something I had noticed in the writing of Hemingway—the patron saint of outdoors writers. In *For Whom the Bell Tolls,* the image of Robert Jordan's goat cheese sandwich with thick slices of onion and crusty bread makes a conversation about love, women, and war both sensual and unforgettable. Equally memorable is the blunt food critique offered by Agustín, his flinty comrade-in-arms, who warns, "You will have a breath that will carry through the forest to the fascists."

Taking a leaf from Papa Hemingway, I have always slipped some food into my fishing-and-hunting stories—even if it's just a Baby Ruth or a piece of my mom's rugelach. Juxtapose that with fishing for largemouth bass in the Everglades and it really hits home with the reader.

You might say that paragraphs about chefs and recipes are not the most obvious fit for magazine pieces about fishing holes and duck blinds, but isn't it all about food? Fishing, hunting, and eating all stem from the same drive: to consume and survive. It seemed like the most natural thing in the world to combine the two. The editors of *Field & Stream, Sports Afield,* and *Outdoor Life* didn't seem to mind one bit.

Half in jest, I introduced myself to my new readers at *New York* by writing, "There is a thing I call Kaminsky's Constant: namely if a man lives long enough, eats long enough, and drinks long enough, there comes a time, usually in his early forties, when his age, waistline, and IQ are the same number."

I wrote that *half* in jest. The other half . . . Well, that's my occupational hazard and what prompted me to write this book.

As the Underground Gourmet, I indulged my passion, first developed in two years behind the wheel of a Yellow Cab, for what I call "drive-by dining": a sense of food radar that told me when a place was worth a meal. If a restaurant smelled good, I was interested. Busyness was another good character reference. The real secret—which I sensed years before I could ever verbalize it—was that if the people who worked in the restaurant looked like they actually *enjoyed* doing what they were doing, then they were doing something right. A sour-faced staff is like a six-story Jumbotron flashing "Eat Here At Your Peril!"

At least three times a week, I would grab whoever wanted to join me and head out for the wilds of Queens, the shores of Staten Island, the back alleys of Brooklyn, the northernmost reaches of the Bronx, the forgotten ethnic enclaves of Manhattan, searching out the best food in town, whether it was Italian, Jewish, Chinese, Korean, Mexican, Russian, German, Greek, Indian, Persian, Vietnamese, Spanish, Dominican, Peruvian, Japanese, Lebanese, Turkish, Cuban, Polish, Hungarian, Portuguese, or Norwegian. Ethiopian too. Also Palestinian, Uzbeki, West Indian, Puerto Rican, to name just a few.

Did I mention that New York is the greatest restaurant town on earth? We may not have an indigenous cuisine, unless you count dirty-water hot dogs, but we sure have the cultural critical mass for an amazing variety of ethnic cuisine. A food critic could not ask for more.

In an interview with Dick Cavett, Bette Davis once confessed that she had been a virgin until she was twenty-eight years old, explaining that, once she had taken the plunge, she did everything in her power to make up for lost time. As covering the New York food world became my occupation, I was as eager as Bette to experience more. Within two years I had put on fifteen pounds. But I was having too good a time to pay attention to hazards—occupational or otherwise.

Writing about food for *New York* also gave me entrée into the world of celebrity chefs. I had cornered the admittedly small market for seven-thousand-word cover pieces on significant restaurant openings. When Daniel Boulud or Alain Ducasse or Thomas Keller opened a place aiming at four stars from the *New York Times,* I got to be the fly on the wall reporting on the frenzied critical path that climaxed on Opening Day. I traveled to France with Daniel Boulud on what I came to think of as The 100,000 Calorie Tour. My immediate purpose was to see the farm where he grew up, meet his family, and have a Sunday dinner. His goal was to introduce his young wine director Jean-Luc

Le Dû to the greatest winemakers in Burgundy and the Rhône Valley. We drank absurdly great wine and ate enough foie gras to endanger Europe's goose population.

When café society's headquarters, Le Cirque, closed up shop for a year while preparing for a move to new quarters, I went to France and Italy with owner Sirio Maccioni and his band of chefs—submitting, in the name of accurate reportage, to an unending movable feast. For the record, I also shucked oysters, peeled and sectioned lemons, and sliced potatoes. I like the camaraderie of the kitchen.

Once you forge an acquaintance with chefs and devote yourself to the intricacies of how they think and cook, it's not too long before you get invited to collaborate with them on that rite of passage: the Very Pretty Coffee Table Cookbook. I worked for four years on *The Elements of Taste* with Gray Kunz, presiding wizard at the revered Lespinasse in the St. Regis Hotel. For nearly a decade Lespinasse captured top honors citywide and nationwide for Kunz's exquisite and eclectic cuisine. Our concept was simple: to analyze all foods and the way that chefs compose recipes, with the same rigor that wine writers use to describe just one food, fermented grape juice. We came up with twenty-two elements of taste, but simplified and pared the number down to fourteen when *Food & Wine* editor in chief Dana Cowin told us it was too complicated, bordering on geekiness.

If Gray Kunz was the alpha of my cookbook career, the omega was the corresponding collection of tailgating recipes that I wrote with football legend and commentator John Madden. This involved traveling coast to coast, to every parking lot in the NFL where tailgating was allowed, walking up and down endless rows of pickup trucks, inviting myself to other people's parties. I ate my way through a button-popping menu of venison chilies, taco salads, hot dogs, sausages, and Jell-O shots, about which I can report that the effect of a two-ounce cube of grape Jell-O laced with vodka is indistinguishable from a tab of purple Owsley. Among my rewards, I found the best barbecued brisket in America (it was made by the McSparin brothers in Parking Lot G, Arrowhead Stadium, at every Kansas City Chiefs home game).

There was a schizophrenic aspect to working on these two cookbooks at the same time as I saw one morning when I finished the reporting for the Gray Kunz recipe for "Braised Short Ribs with Pickled Papaya and Horseradish." This was without question his most complicated dish, consisting of thirty-one ingredients and featuring a spice rub, a marinade, a braising liquid, and a parallel pickling operation, all of which took place over the course of three days. I was noting down how long to pan-roast the coriander seeds in the spice rub when Madden's agent, Sandy Montag, called.

"I have Madden on the line. He's going to Vegas for a few days and will be hard to reach. If you have any questions, ask them now."

I looked through my notes. "Coach," I said, using the title that comes naturally to anyone who works with John, "I need to go over the recipe for the whole sirloin." I was referring to a fifteen-pound piece of meat that he had grilled expertly.

"Well, you take a sirloin and you salt and pepper it, maybe some garlic salt too. Then you cook it for . . ." He raised his voice as he questioned his wife: "Hey, Virginia, that whole sirloin—what do you cook it for? Two or three hours?"

Then, turning back to the phone: "You cook it two or three hours."

As I later realized in the course of writing two grilling books, Madden's advice, though deceptively simple, makes good kitchen sense: big pieces of meat take a long time, and there is no strict rule to timing; you cook it until it's done.

Through the Madden and Kunz projects, I learned that the thing about cookbooks is that you don't write them so much as eat your way through them. You cook and sample recipes, dipping your index finger into sauces and fillings and frostings, constantly tasting and retasting. And you're doing it during work hours, not at mealtime. It's a hazardous lifestyle. I didn't know that when I started, but I noticed, at the end of the Madden project, that the Carhartt overalls that I wore to places like Green Bay, Wisconsin, bulged in the middle, a reflection of my growing girth. I consoled myself with the words of P. G. Wodehouse: "Boys have stomachs. Men have bellies."

By that measure, I was becoming quite a man.

Another hazardous perk of food-writerdom was an unsolicited nine- or ten-course tasting menu that dogged me whenever I visited a restaurant where I knew the chef or, at least, someone on the staff recognized me. "The chef would like to make a menu for you," the waiter would say with a wink-wink leer. It is hard to complain about being force-fed a mind-blowing array of dishes, especially when envious diners at other tables must content themselves with the everyday menu. But the truth of the matter is this omnivore's nirvana is not achieved painlessly. There always comes a time in such meals when the chef will send out a surprise of foie gras or squab right after I have polished off what I thought was a concluding course of beef. In such instances I will often run up the white flag and instruct the waiter, "Please, tell the chef he wins."

Lest you think that my new vocation was all a mix of trendy ethnic food from the Outer Boroughs and truffle-showered lark's tongues served up by Manhattan dining divinities, I also came across strange new foods in the course of journalistic assignments around the world. I ate salmon eye—traditionally reserved for honored guests—by the shores of a Finnish lake; grasshoppers at a Zapotec market in Oaxaca; unsightly if delicious corn smut among the Mixtecs of Mitla; *mopane* worms the size of gnocchi at a banquet with the Shona tribespeople of Zimbabwe; barbecued bear ribs brought to me by a California bow hunter who looked a bit like a bear himself; saliva-fermented *chicha* (a beer-like beverage) in a small Inca village in the Peruvian highlands; prairie oysters (cattle testicles) in Livingston, Montana; alligator tail batter-fried by Jimmy Tiger, a Miccosukee hunter in the Everglades; and roasted dwarf armadillo that two young boys in Uruguay delivered to my hotel after a chance early-morning conversation about the local hunting. Equally exotic to me, fried Spam, presented to me by a family of walleye anglers at the Red Squirrel Lodge in Bemidji, Minnesota, where, in a ritual to mark the opening of fishing season, the least successful angler of the day is required/honored to eat a plateful of this all-American "delicacy."

After another five years of magazine and newspaper writing, cookbook work, and tasting menus, I had acquired an additional fifteen pounds. My heart, my gut, and my blood sugar were unimpressed by the four-star pedigree of many of those extra calories. To them, there was no distinction between a Ferran Adrià tasting menu and a Colonel Sanders Variety Bucket.

As a matter of pure economics, I couldn't afford to give too much thought to the toll my new career was taking on my body. My job was my diet, and my diet consisted of eating, tasting, enjoying, and reporting on the best, most interesting meals I could find. Under such work rules, it's a given that you will sacrifice some health considerations.

The day I turned fifty, I filmed a show for the Food Network in Oaxaca, Mexico. In honor of this milestone, and since I was the producer and got to call the shots, I ordered up a sheep roast and invited a whole village where mescal was made. The local band, undeterred by their inability to agree on a key in which they could all play, serenaded me with a joyful, though barely recognizable, rendition of "Happy Birthday." A fun day, but not a slimming one.

My waistline creep continued: from size thirty-four in my early thirties to "thirty-eight" as I crossed the Big Five-Oh. Note: I put the thirty-eight in quotes because it is usually a fiction, representing an imaginary line that few men like to admit they have crossed. On the other side of thirty-eight lies forty, which begins with "f," which stands for "fat." As long as a man can keep size thirty-eight-inch pants buttoned, even if he needs to draw a deep breath to do so, he can tell himself that he is not borderline obese. No delusion hangs by more slender threads.

Then my doctor told me I needed to go on Lipitor.

No problem. I began taking the drug, which I dismissively referred to as "my cheese license."

I was less lighthearted when my nephews began referring to me—and my stomach—as "the Buddha." I gave in to my wife's advice and began going to the gym. Although I have always walked a lot (the norm in NYC), waded miles of rivers while trout fishing, and biked around Prospect Park for years, I regarded gyms as the realm of garish spandex outfits and unmanly group calisthenics to the beat of an annoying tape loop . . . probably Abba.

To my surprise, I liked working out, especially under the tutelage of a great trainer (have you ever met anyone who didn't think his trainer or shrink was great?).

Soon I felt better, but fitness training plus food writing, and all the eating that it entailed, still equaled fat.

"You have to do something about your weight," said my doctor, Steve Tay.

"Hey, I eat healthy and exercise," I answered, as if good intentions ever scored a victory over arterial plaque and elevated blood sugar.

My protests notwithstanding, my weight curve went in only one direction as I aged. I wasn't John Candy fat, maybe more like Seth Rogen pudgy. But, as I learned the day my life-insurance renewal was denied, you don't have to be a super-fat boy to be a candidate for heart disease and diabetes. I am far from alone in this risk pool. The fastest-growing life-threatening condition among Americans is obesity, going from one-in-six fifteen years ago to one-in-four today. In the South the trend is to one-in-three.

When I was told that my weight was a possible precursor of diabetes, I permanently disabled the snooze setting on my life's alarm clock. I want to see my kids get married and watch my grandchildren grow. I want to fish the Missouri River in my eighties. Most of all, I want to stick around and enjoy the senses of taste and smell that I was born with: more great wine, more juicy steaks on the Patagonian plains. But how does a guy who loves food and wine—in fact, makes his living writing about them—gain control of what he puts in his body?

Tens of millions of Americans face a similar dilemma. Nobody wants to stop enjoying food, but neither does anybody want to lop 20 percent off his or her anticipated life span. I could have responded to Dr. Steve's admonition with the words of one of my food-writing heroes, A. J. Liebling of *The New Yorker,* who wrote in his mouth-watering memoir *Between Meals,* "No sane man can afford to dispense with debilitating pleasures; no ascetic can be considered reliably sane."

If you follow Liebling's go-to-hell approach to weight control, you will surely have some memorable meals, but it is cold comfort—like graveyard-cold—if, as Liebling did, you end up weighing three hundred–plus pounds and dropping dead at age fifty-nine. A much better model, who writes about food with equal brio, is Calvin Trillin, also of *The New Yorker.* When I asked him his secret for weight control, he credited his late wife: "When Alice was alive, if I had to sum up my wife's method of keeping my weight down in one word, I'd say 'nagging' would be that word, sometimes leavened by ridicule." He left out that the bicycle is his preferred method of transport in Manhattan. I have both a wife and a bike; so, if Trillin could do it, I could do it too.

I took my doctor's advice seriously. I didn't stop drinking, but no more than two glasses of wine at dinner was my goal. White bread, white rice, and white potatoes were put on the "No Eat" list. I became more diligent about exercise, but I had been training for years, so that side of the equation didn't require as much reprogramming as my diet.

After six months of discipline (during which time I went to South America for extended stays to research a cookbook featuring grilled meat and red wine), I melted away twenty-five pounds (and another fifteen since then). More to the point of this book, I have not put them back on.

As Steve foretold, my blood sugar came down, and as my insurance agent promised, my policy was approved. The guy who had been fat at fifty was now slimmer at sixty. I have changed what I eat and how much I eat, and the same goes for drink. It has become second nature to take the stairs leading to my apartment two at a time. I thought those days were long past. My suit size has gone down, my shirts are three sizes smaller at the neck, my XL tees have gone from too tight to too big, and it is no longer hard to breathe when I bend over to tie my shoes. Once again, I have a thirty-four-inch waistline, the size I wore just before I became a professional eater.

I didn't know it at the time, but, instinctively, I was putting Culinary Intelligence into practice. Please take note: I didn't say Culinary Super-Intelligence. It's not astrophysics. My approach is much more practical than it is intellectual. It starts from the premise that anyone who wants to eat a healthy diet is confronted by a big obstacle: a food culture based on industrially processed ingredients and the unholy trinity of sugar, salt, and fat, all used to boost flavor and create pleasing texture. Getting people to eat fattening fast food, made hyper-palatable with chemically enhanced ingredients, is like giving candy to a baby. Without thinking, the baby eats it.

Step one on the path to Culinary Intelligence is to break this habit of mindless eating and to cut out processed foods. Do it now. You will lose weight.

But if you give something up, how do you replace it? To begin with, eat fresh, peak-flavor ingredients that a caveman—or at least a farmer from a few thousand years ago—might have recognized as food. A delicious melon, crisp and sweet sugar snap peas, or a golden-brown oven-roasted free-range chicken doesn't need very much in the way of sugar, salt, or added fat. Do healthy ingredients cost more? Sometimes, but not always, particularly when they are local and in season.

In *Blue Trout and Black Truffles,* a lyric and nostalgic memoir of food and dining in Europe before and immediately after World War II, *New Yorker* contributor Joseph Wechsberg credited

Charles Gundel, a Budapest restaurateur of the early twentieth century, with the following: "It is difficult to make something good out of second-class materials, but it is quite easy to spoil the first-class ones." So, yes, you need the best ingredients you can afford, but, just as important, whoever is making the food in your household must know what to do with them in order to coax out the most satisfying flavor and texture. A bad cook can mess up the most costly ingredients. A good one can make them heavenly.

In a restaurant you rely on the chef, although more than one chef has resorted to shock-and-awe amounts of butter and salt to liven up a recipe. At home these decisions fall to the cook-in-residence. If you are that person, you need to understand flavor and how to prepare food that is satisfying without making you fat. Take-out food won't do the trick. Nor will a steady diet of ready-made meals. Good cooking with real ingredients is the only way to eat a healthy, satisfying diet. Some authorities may not be so insistent on this point. I see no other way.

You may be tempted to say that my perspective is not applicable to the rest of the country because I live in food-crazed New York, and, more particularly, in Brooklyn, where the food-and-restaurant scene is arguably the most vibrant in the city. To me Brooklyn is a magical place where old-time ethnic-food stores abound: where butchers, greengrocers, and cheese shops are on every street, and where, in recent years, there has been an explosion of farmers' markets, farm-to-table restaurants, and urban farms on rooftops and street corners. My Brooklyn feels more like a village or small American town from years gone by than suburban America, where I spent my childhood.

This is not to say that America is all malls and McDonald's. One recent Thanksgiving, we found great heritage-breed turkeys in my wife's hometown, Rockford, Illinois. I have bought beautiful local vegetables in the Winn-Dixie Supermarket in Boynton Beach, Florida. In season you can find local and organic products at farmstands and, increasingly, in supermarkets just about everywhere. Moreover, such staples as beans, chickpeas, lentils, anchovies, sardines, and high-quality canned, bottled, or frozen vegetables are not difficult to buy in any supermarket anytime. I once made a whole seven-course meal according to the recipes of a demanding French chef by creatively substituting with ingredients from the Grand Union in Lake Placid, New York.

Often overlooked—but they shouldn't be, because they are no longer confined to big cities—are ethnic markets. As more of our crops are grown and harvested by these new Americans, there are more markets that cater to them. In these stores, you will undoubtedly find a lot of unprocessed "real" ingredients. Latin and Asian markets are always a good bet.

So, yes, on any given day, I suppose Brooklynites may have more access to a greater variety of the best ingredients than people in Duluth or Tallahassee. But you can eat well and healthfully everywhere if you apply your inborn Culinary Intelligence.

Ten words tell the CI story:

Buy the best ingredients you can afford. Cook them well.

If you are not gifted in the kitchen, you can add twelve more words: live with someone who likes to cook and is good at it.

If your goal is to adopt a diet that works for the rest of your life, always remember, eating should be a pleasure, and not a penance for the environmental and economic sins of our times. So, although I responded seriously to my insurance-flunking wake-up call, being serious did not need to mean somber or joyless. But then, we are a country with a long-standing, often religious distrust of pleasure. Since food brings pleasure, it also invites sermonizing. Whether we celebrate the virtues of free-range and local ingredients or excoriate the malefactors of Big Agriculture, the argument can sometimes veer into a level of sobriety that takes the fun out of food. Eating local and thinking global; banning genetically modified food; curtailing the excesses of factory farming that condemn millions of animals to nasty, brutish, and short lives; confronting the tsunami of marketing, packaging, and advertising that, in the space of fifteen years, has seduced average Americans into consuming three hundred more calories per day and collectively putting on two billion pounds of body weight—all of these are pressing social and moral issues, but not particularly helpful in choosing your next meal.

You and I are not a social issue. We are individual human beings who consume food in order to stay alive. Statistics don't decide to eat a healthier diet; individuals do. Consider this: everyone who lost weight over the last twenty years of a steadily fattening America did so in spite of statistics. Forget the trend lines—which are alarming—and think about yourself.

The Most Important Thing: Flavor per Calorie

If I had to reduce Culinary Intelligence to one guiding principle, it would be maximizing Flavor per Calorie (FPC): the notion that if ingredients are chosen on the basis of optimum flavor, and prepared with the goal of intensifying that flavor, then you can be satisfied while eating less.

It is important to understand that taste starts in the mouth but does not end there. You have five different kinds of taste receptors on your palate. As I learned from Charles S. Zuker, whose groundbreaking work in the science of taste has provided the first full exploration of our principal taste receptors, some of them are also found in your gastrointestinal tract.

Clearly, you don't taste with your stomach the way that you do with your mouth. Your palate is a gateway. It is designed to discern different tastes so that you can avoid harmful or nutritionally worthless substances and consume nourishing ones. After food has passed through this portal, the next line of taste receptors, in your stomach, signals your body that it is receiving nutrients. By maximizing FPC, the stomach you have pampered with great flavor will receive a return message from the brain: "We're cool. I've had enough."

It stands to reason, then, that if you get more taste bang for the bite, you won't need so many bites. If, on the other hand, your food is indifferently prepared from ingredients that lack flavor, the only alternative is to pile on the high-caloric combo of sugar, salt, and fat.

Achieving maximum Flavor per Calorie starts with ingredients as they come from nature. For fruits, ripeness is paramount. For vegetables, freshness. The flavor of meat, fish, and poultry depends on what the animal ate, how it lived (was it free-range or confined?), how long it lived (was it long enough to develop marbling?). Was it cured or aged afterward?

If ingredients start out full-flavored, then realizing much of their FPC potential will result from further developing flavor through cooking. Caramelizing vegetables and creating a crunchy browned crust on meats are key techniques. So are long, slow braises that tenderize meat and help develop the mysterious but essential "Fifth Taste" known as umami, often described as "deliciousness" (see page 122).

My approach to all food is that of a sensualist, not a Trappist monk. I believe in gratification, not denial. To illustrate this, let's put aside, for the moment, the question of fresh, locally grown fruits and vegetables versus out-of-season produce from distant places. (I'm in favor of the former and not so much the latter.) Let's consider, instead, some foods that are not commonly found in many weight-control plans: beer, steak, chocolate, and cheese. I enjoy them—perhaps not in the quantities that I once did, but I found that I didn't have to give them up so long as I sprang for the best products I could find.

Try this experiment yourself: side by side, taste a Coors Light and, say, a Dogfish Head 90 Minute India Pale Ale. The advertisements for light beer suggest that you can drink more of it. I should hope so, because one light beer is never going to satisfy you. So, after downing one, you still want more beer-ness. You're a little bit more full after two beers, but still there is something lacking, so you pop-top beer number three.

This could go on for a while, but no matter how many light beers you drink you will feel shortchanged in the beer satisfaction department. On the other hand, with the India Pale Ale—it doesn't have to be India Pale Ale, just a real, full-flavored, full-calorie beer—you're going to get that yeasty, fizzy smell, bubbles that jab your tongue with force rather than teeny pops, and a sharpness that can cut through the richness of the most succulent meat while it refreshes your palate. Even the beer belch of the India Pale is going to taste more like beer when it comes up than the Coors Light did going down. Granted, one or two India Pales aren't going to get you as hammered as a six-pack of Coors Light, but for pure taste satisfaction, the full-on real brew will win every time.

Or take the case of grass-fed versus grain-fed beef. Americans have been brought up to prefer super-tender, mild-tasting, corn-fed beef. This has been very good for the corn business. But cattle evolved to eat grass, not corn. My experience over the last twenty-five years, when visiting Argentina and Uruguay, gave me an appreciation of the deeper flavor of grass-fed animals. Their meat tastes more beefy, even wild. I sometimes wondered, was I simply selling myself on grass-fed because I was ideologically attached to the concept of livestock eating their original state-of-nature diet?

To put my belief to the test, I arranged a series of blind tastings with my friends Frank Castronovo and Frank Falcinelli, the proprietors of Frankies Spuntino and Prime Meats, two very popular restaurants near my home. The Franks, as they are known in the hood, are Italian Americans from Queens who grew up playing street hockey together and later apprenticed under two of Europe's greatest chefs—Paul Bocuse and André Daguin—before reuniting as restaurateurs twenty years later.

At each of our tasting sessions, a group of seven people in the food world (chefs, writers, my wife and daughter, two NYU grad students) sampled beef from seven of the top artisanal producers in the country. We tried rib eyes and strip steaks, also known as "New York cuts" or "shell steaks," fourteen pieces of beef in all. The clear favorite—five first-place votes and two seconds—was a grass-fed, dry-aged rib eye from Rosenkranz Farms in the Finger Lakes (via New York purveyor DeBragga). Grass-fed beef has more FPC, and, in my experience, you will need to eat less of it in order to be satisfied. The other moral is that, just as with great wine, good meat will develop more complex flavors as it ages.

Continue this experiment and try some high-quality dark chocolate alongside a Hershey bar. I find that a two-inch square of Scharffen Berger 70% gets my taste buds firing in a way that a whole Hershey bar never does (NB: Hershey owns the Scharffen Berger brand). Likewise, a one-ounce piece of artisanal Vermont cow's-milk cheese that tastes like a French Tomme lights my fire much more than some "zesty" house-brand pepper jack. Beware of the word "zesty": it's marketese for "doctored up with lots of chemicals that you won't notice because it's also really spicy."

Insisting on fuller-flavored ingredients is sometimes faulted as elitist. This is phony populist logic. Fruits and vegetables in season are comparatively less expensive than produce that comes from the other side of the continent, or the world. Factory-farmed meat, fish, and poultry are less expensive, if less flavorful, than prime ingredients, but their deficiencies can be cheaply doctored up with crispy breadings and sweet, gloppy sauces. Moreover, when you factor in agricultural subsidies, fast food actually costs more for each unit of flavor per calorie than we pay for unadulterated, old-fashioned ingredients. If you shop intelligently and seasonally, and prepare more of the food you eat, the hit to your wallet is certainly not more and probably less.

Furthermore, in a country approaching a 40-percent rate of obesity, it is not unreasonable to argue that health-care costs more than offset any pennies that may be saved on inferior products.

I have been lucky that my profession has taken me around the country, and the world, driving home the lesson that our conventional, convenience-food diet is not the only way to get your daily sustenance. In my travels, I have been welcomed into the kitchens of many gifted chefs, some of them famous and more of them not well known beyond the family table. They have taught me most of what I know about what makes food delicious. Applying those lessons enabled me to make adjustments in how I eat without sacrificing pleasure. There are many ways to enhance the joy of eating—some of them fattening, but many of them not.

For a change in diet to succeed, it must be at least as satisfying as the unhealthful fast food and processed ingredients that it replaces. The only way I know to achieve this is through maximizing Flavor per Calorie. It is my guide to deriving as much pleasure from food as I did in the days when I ate and drank without giving much thought to health implications. I am no less a hedonist now, but a slimmer and fitter one.

CHAPTER II Mind over Midsection

Nobody wants to be overweight, yet more and more of us are. Why do we eat in a way that produces results so contrary to our wishes? I think the answer lies in the brain. It reacts to hunger pangs and then makes a decision: eat something that will satisfy, the quicker the better. Long-term nutritional sense rarely figures into this process. You're hungry; you eat. For many it's a never-changing one-act play performed daily, usually resulting in a lifetime of putting on weight. In my case, for nearly thirty years, the narrative was the following:

STOMACH: I'm hungry.

RIGHT BRAIN: I want pizza!

LEFT BRAIN: No way. It's fattening.

RIGHT BRAIN: Just one little piece, okay?

LEFT BRAIN: Then will you stop pestering me?

RIGHT BRAIN: I promise.

Walk to pizza parlor. Order and pay for slice. Right hand brings a slice of pizza to mouth. Mouth bites off a piece, chews, and swallows. The pizza is warm, crisp, melty, salty, and bright with tomato flavor.

STOMACH: Man, that was good!

RIGHT BRAIN: You bet. How about another?

LEFT BRAIN: Hold on. We had a deal.

RIGHT BRAIN AND STOMACH (IN UNISON): Shut up!

Left hand reaches into blue-jeans pocket, retrieves some singles, tells pizza guy to keep the change. Once again right hand brings pizza to mouth. Another shipment heads south.

RIGHT BRAIN: How did I let that happen? I hate myself!

LEFT BRAIN: That makes two of us.

Sound familiar? Resolving such conflicts, understanding what you need in terms of sustenance versus what you have become conditioned to want, is at the heart of CI. It's a simple proposition, but complicated in terms of the biology and psychology that underlie what and why we eat.

I think that, to a certain degree, the media, the food industry, and many nutrition experts have burdened us with a too simplistic and incomplete paradigm about the nature of food. The body is thought of as a machine, and food as nothing more than fuel with some engine additives that lubricate the parts and keep the pipes clean.

This outlook encourages us to understand food as a collection of simpler chemical components rather than extremely complex organic substances. But looking at nutrients in isolation—which is what so many studies and diets do—is like removing all the notes from a musical score, putting them in a box, shaking the box, pouring the notes on a table, and hoping that they land in exactly the same order as Beethoven's Piano Sonata No. 28 in A major.

Life is never that simple. Adding broccoli to your diet because some study said it fights cancer; cutting down on one kind of fat because a lab rat ate itself to death on a diet of lamb liver; consuming expensive four-ounce containers of yogurt in hopes that its bacteria will bless you with the life span of a redwood tree are not realistic hopes. Nothing you put in your body has just one effect. Everything is multifaceted and interrelated. A diet of whole foods has all the nutrients we need.

Supplements won't make up for the deficiencies that come with a processed-food diet, but they will generate *mucho dinero* for the supplement industry. Still, we go on spending enormous sums on protein powders, herbal supplements, vitamins, minerals, nutrient extracts, all of them ripped from their natural context, where they are elements of much more complex foods. For this reason, many scientists believe that a simple pill or powder won't do the trick. Every food is more than the sum of its nutrients. The balance and interaction of nutrients are what make them beneficial.

Nutritionally speaking, it's time to jettison the fuel-and-engine metaphor in favor of one that views everything that lives as its own complex ecosystem. Your particular ecosystem consists of a community of trillions of living cells. So does the diet that sustains it. It is the product of evolution. This brings me to the question of what is a "natural diet," how did it evolve, and do we all have to eat like Neanderthals? Among advocates of different diets, much is made of what our earliest ancestors supposedly ate. The implication is that if we were to eat the same way, we would all have washboard abs. The theory is that before culture and technology entered the picture, humans ate foods that were naturally good.

But good for what? We evolved to live just long enough to guarantee that a sufficient number of our kids reached the age of prime reproductive and child-caring potential. In other words, our ancestral diet gave us the best chance to reach a life span of thirty-something.

Although childhood obesity is a growing problem, it's not those first thirty years that concern most of us so much as the forty or fifty that follow. That's where bad habits take their inevitable toll. Evolution tells us little more than how our distant ancestors adapted to maximize their nutritional opportunities. Obesity was not a big problem. The nutritional requirements of human beings remained the same for ten thousand generations of hunting and gathering. Compare that with the five hundred generations or so that followed the invention of agriculture, and only two or three generations since the adoption of industrially processed foods and the widespread availability of fat, sugar, and salt.

No matter how sophisticated we may have become as gourmets, food remains a basic need. We all have food cravings, and among the most fundamental of them are those for sugar, salt, and fat. There is good reason for this: these nutrients are crucial to maintaining good health. But we don't need them all the time, or in a form that goes straight to the bloodstream and, from there, takes up residence as fat in potbellies and clogged arteries.

A word or two here in defense of dietary fat. It is a fact of evolution that without increased fat consumption our ancient relatives would never have developed large brains. According to the prevailing theory, when humanity's birthplace in East Africa dried out, about two and a half million years ago, one group of prehuman apes moved toward a diet of large quantities of fibrous food that we would find largely indigestible. These long-extinct cousins of ours developed huge, heavily muscled jaws and molars and Klingon-like brows to anchor their chewing muscles. Big brows, big jaws, small brains.

Our branch of the family tree responded to the change in the environment by adopting a diet that was energy-dense, containing more animal protein and fat. These not-yet-human primates required food more like that of carnivores and less like the diet of their plant-dependent cousins. They needed meat, for the energy and body-building qualities of protein and for the high concentration of stored energy in fat. Both are necessary for development of the brain, a ravenous energy-consumer that accounts for about 27 percent of our total energy expenditure.

Many anthropologists believe that the story of human evolution—basically, a tale of apes with big brains—is inextricably bound up with the taming of fire and the advent of cooking. Some scientists, notably Richard Wrangham of Harvard, take the argument even further. Cooking, he maintains, was the key advance that led to the tremendous gains in brainpower that distinguished the genus *Homo* from the less clever creatures whose branches withered off our family tree.

When our forebears ate cooked meat, less energy was required for digestion. They evolved a smaller digestive tract. Cooking took up the workload needed to meet the requirements of a bigger brain. Had we stayed with the fruits-and-shoots diets of the other apes, we would probably have the brains of chimps. This raises an interesting point: will we revert to knuckle-walking dim-wittedness if we all eat low-fat vegetarian diets?

Fat is good, just not so much of it, and certainly not the hard trans fats that clog arteries. Fear of fat has driven us to consume great quantities of processed carbohydrates, which the body converts to sugar and—ironically—deposits as unhealthy amounts of fat.

The reason we crave fat so strongly, along with salt and sugar, is that the human appetite evolved in response to the scarcity of these vital nutrients that often confronted hunter-gatherers. There were times when game was scarce, drought and floods destroyed fruits and vegetables, and salt licks were few and far between. Our genes do not yet recognize that we are living in what Paleolithic people would have thought of as a permanent best-case scenario: salt, sugar, and fat are all around us in health-threatening superabundance, so there is no need to gorge on them today because they might disappear tomorrow. Maybe in another fifty thousand years, natural selection will produce human beings who crave whole grains, high-fiber vegetables, and unfried chicken. For now, though, inside every one of us is a prehistoric person fearful of starving on an ice age tundra.

Our food culture, with the billions upon billions of dollars it generates, is built on a foundation of fulfilling our Cro-Magnon cravings, packaging and repackaging the trifecta of sugar, salt, and fat. In present-day America, if you want to eat a healthy diet, the only way to do it is to find your own alternative path to equal satisfaction. This always requires giving up or curtailing some foods to which we have grown accustomed. So, although the word "Don't!" is not a sustainable long-term eating plan, it is often the only way to begin to make the transition to better, though still pleasurable, nutrition. It will take off weight, and that fact alone is often sufficient to help us get on track.

Making a few immediate changes is a lot easier than daily calorie counting, predetermined menu plans, or overloading on one food—whether it's grapefruit, seaweed, eggs, or steak. Such strategies are untenable over the long run. They require you to be on duty all the time, but that is not the way to get pleasure out of your meals. To eat well, you need to relax and enjoy.

If, in the beginning, you merely stop eating certain fattening foods, you won't have to obsess over how many calories there are in every bite of every meal. This doesn't mean that you can never have a pastry again, just not every day.

Mostly, what you need to do is to seek out satisfaction in new, sometimes different ways. You know and I know that no one is going to be satisfied replacing a cheeseburger with a bowl of boiled chickpeas. But if you add a cup of white wine to the cooking liquid and some oven-roasted tomatoes, fresh herbs, a lashing of good vinegar, a bit of crunchy flaky salt, and a drizzle of fresh floral olive oil, you now have a delicious and appetizing nonburger.

Any change in diet requires close attention in the beginning. Then, like any acquired skill, new choices become second nature and you hardly have to think about them, but you must stay in practice. Because we live in what Kelly Brownell of the Rudd Center for Food Policy and Obesity has called "a toxic food environment," it is easy to be overweight. All over the world, traditional diets are being replaced by high-fat fast foods, sugar-sweetened beverages, and simple carbohydrates, usually in the form of refined white flour.

Barry Popkin, a professor at the University of North Carolina, is one of the leading experts on this dietary transformation, known as "the nutrition transition." He told me that, in the last sixty years, as soft drinks, burgers, fries, and snack foods were adopted all around the world, there has not been a single example—not one—of any developed nation reducing the number of people who are overweight. We are awash in a sea of empty calories. In a world where famine still commands more attention than obesity, it may come as a surprise that the more pervasive scourge turns out to be overeating—or, more precisely, eating too much of the wrong stuff. There are almost a billion and a half overweight people in the world, nearly twice as many as the underweight figure of eight hundred million.

There is very little mystery about what dietary demons produced this result. They are ubiquitous, and if you do nothing more than stop consuming them you will be taking a big step toward a more healthful diet. You will weigh less and feel better too.

No White Stuff

The first piece of diet advice I received turned out to be the best, or at least the most immediately effective. Without it I wouldn't have taken off those initial pounds so quickly, and without that encouragement I would not have followed through for nearly ten years and counting. It was given to me by Barry Zins, the fellow who sold me life insurance after I flunked one physical, took off weight, and then passed another. Barry, apart from being a nice guy, had a financial stake in getting me across the life-insurance finish line, and, like me, he happened to have high blood sugar.

"Cut out the white food," he said.

The No White Stuff rule is not news to you if you read diet books or fitness magazines that promise "The Fast Track to Bed-Busting Abs." But I don't. I thought I was doing the right thing, going out of my way to avoid fats and exercising regularly, but my weight kept going up. Barry's low-carb No White Stuff regimen was new and surprising information.

I turned to him and said, "Huh?"

"White flour, white sugar, white rice, and potatoes. They turn to fat more quickly."

"Surely you don't mean no pasta?" I protested. Like many who endured the last thirty years of fat phobia, I thought that a diet with lots of pasta was a great way to get protein while steering clear of cholesterol-raising meat.

"Whole-grain pasta is fine," Barry said. "But stay off the white flour."

Whole-grain is an important aspect of any serious attempt to take weight off and keep it off. The science behind this is pretty simple. Refined flour—that is, grain that has had its outer shell removed—is quite easy for the human digestive tract to break down into sugar. It is not the sugar per se that is harmful, but the rate of absorption. The fiber in whole grains slows this process down. The surge in blood sugar when there is no mediating fiber kicks off a biological chain of events, stimulating insulin and eventually ending up as fat.

Taking the whole-grain plunge was a big step. In my brother Bob's words, I disparaged whole-grain products as "pine-bark mulch." When my mother-in-law, Gini, baked us multigrain bread during our visits to her home in Rockford, Illinois, I begged my wife to find us something other than "Mom's torture bread." Ditto for whole-grain muffins, pie crusts, and cookies. I was convinced that whole grains were in the same category as cod-liver oil: reputedly good for you because they're unpleasurable. If I needed any more confirmation, there were all those floss-defying grain bits that lodge between your teeth.

I have since changed my haughty attitude toward whole grains.

Actually, I have come to prefer dark bread and adore whole-grain flatbreads and crackers. If you make the whole-grain switch, please read the label before buying multigrain bread. No doubt the package will be emblazoned with health claims—which always seem to come with exclamation points—but if you take the time to read the label, the first ingredient often says white or wheat flour. Maybe it will have the qualifiers "unbleached" or "organic," but it's still processed flour. I keep shopping until I find bread whose first listed ingredient is a whole grain. Sometimes there is no way around settling for bread that has some white flour, in which case just make sure it's not the first ingredient listed.

I will not attempt to argue that whole-grain pasta slips and slides all over your tongue in the same fun way that white pasta does, but more powerful flavors and different textures in a sauce can compensate for lack of slitheriness. As a side benefit, the pursuit of added flavor led me to consume more grilled vegetables (such as radicchio and zucchini), roast tomatoes, and olives on my pasta. They boost flavor and add interesting texture: more FPC.

A year after reluctantly giving up white pasta, I came across some cheering news. It turns out that not all white pastas are equally bad. Hard durum-semolina wheat—from which the very best Italian pasta is made—is more slowly digested than pasta made from regular refined white flour. It was a great relief to learn, after I went cold-turkey on white flour, that I could have the occasional bowl of traditional pasta without upsetting my body chemistry and heading back down the road of weight gain. When cooked al dente—slightly chewy, which is the only way you should ever cook pasta—it is also more slowly absorbed into the bloodstream, and that means less of a spike in blood sugar.

Potatoes Are White

Potatoes are on the semi-forbidden list because they are high in starch, which the body turns to sugar very quickly. In scientific terms, just like white flour, potatoes have a high glycemic index. This is a measure of how quickly food is converted to sugar in your bloodstream. Foods with a high glycemic index (white bread, for example) boost the sugar levels in your blood, leaving you susceptible to a subsequent sugar crash, which stimulates your hunger so you often eat more and put on more weight. I was not completely surprised when Walter Willett, a Harvard professor and the nation's foremost dietary epidemiologist, told me that potatoes can spike your blood sugar more than pure cane sugar.

Giving up potatoes was not that hard for me: I have always thought of them as something bland to be served alongside more exciting food. But then it hit home that taking the potato pledge meant no more French fries or potato chips. I have never met anyone who does not like French fries or chips. Well, there was one kid, a friend of my younger daughter, Lily, who claimed that she didn't like potato chips except for sour-cream-and-onion-flavored ones, but I think she was just being willful, so I didn't believe her.

You can't almost/kind of/sort of not eat fries and chips the way you can stop after a bite or two of buttered bread. Once you have that first one, you are going to keep eating. Why? Because the combination of saltiness, fattiness, and crispness is super-palatable. Resistance is futile. That's just the nature of potatoes, salt, hot fat, and people. So the way not to have the last one is not to have the first one. If you have the option of requesting "hold the fries," do so. If you must, feel free to steal a couple from your spouse, or your child, either with their permission or when they are not looking.

Avoiding potatoes as a general rule should not be confused with a divinely decreed prohibition. Life has its special occasions, and I am happy to accommodate them. In that regard, one meal in Peru remains particularly vivid. I had taken advantage of an opportunity to see Machu Picchu, which lived up to its reputation for breathtaking beauty. But no one told me about another wonder of the Altiplano: amazing potatoes!

My traveling partner was Doug Rodriguez, a Cuban American chef who has been called the godfather of Nuevo Latino cuisine. Like many of my favorite modern chefs, he has the ability to take traditional cuisine and "gastronomize" it: i.e., use the techniques of the trained restaurant chef to refine and amplify the tastes and textures of a traditional dish. In terms of CI, it is simply a process of pumping up FPC.

Doug was collecting recipes for a magnum opus on South American foods. My role was helping a publicity firm earn its fee. If you are lucky enough to be even a mid-level food celebrity (that means anyone with a byline in a newspaper, magazine, or, nowadays, an online avatar that is followed by more than a hundred people), freebie trips like this come your way.

Upon arriving in Cuzco—elevation 11,200 feet—the capital of the Inca Empire, Doug and I drank a few cups of coca tea, made from the same plant that, in its highly refined form, is the natural source for cocaine. Two thousand years ago, the Nazca people, who preceded the Incas, were well aware that coca helped counteract the effects of altitude.

Invigorated by our tea, Doug and I strolled through the town and, as is quite natural for a food writer and a chef, into the local market, where we came upon a very large woman who wore a burlap apron, her hands and arms covered with brown soil. If asked to describe her, I would say she looked like a giant potato. Ranged around her in burlap sacks, there were more varieties of potatoes than I knew existed. Potatoes with blue flesh, red flesh, golden flesh flecked with crimson veins; big as grapefruits, small as grapes, round, oval, long, stubby—potatopalooza!

We returned to the hotel, and the prospect the next day of a gut-busting Special Dinner from the Most Famous Chef in Town. "Forget the veal Cordon Bleu," we suggested to him, begging off the tired gourmet warhorse that was featured on the menu. "Tomorrow, we want to taste all those potatoes we saw in the market. And, oh yeah, could you do it at Machu Picchu?"

He could, and we feasted on a vertical potato tasting that demonstrated to me that the bland potatoes that I had written off on taste-and-texture grounds bore little resemblance to the delicious and varied spuds we sampled on a terrace overlooking the breathtaking Inca ruins. Come to think of it, perched as we were on the side of a mountain, it was a *very* vertical potato tasting.

Even though potatoes and I have parted ways for the most part, I would gladly repeat that exploit if I had the chance. Culinary Intelligence is a helpful guide, but it wasn't handed down from Mount Sinai. And, speaking of Mount Sinai, I can't foresee ever giving up my annual potato-latkes party.

Do You Really Need Dessert?

I have often wondered why dessert—the sweet course—is served at the end of the meal. This is not the case in every food culture. In some regional Chinese and Indian cuisines, the sweet course may be served first.

I have posed the dessert-as-meal-ender question to many chefs, and the answer, which has never fully satisfied me, is that dessert completes the experience. That's simply a circular-logic way of saying that it comes at the end of the meal because it's the last course.

Laurent Gras, a brilliant chef who in his early twenties was put in command of the kitchens at two of Alain Ducasse's highest-rated restaurants (three Michelin stars for both Louis XV in Monaco and Restaurant Alain Ducasse in Paris), offered an intriguing answer.

"Everyone craves sweetness, but you can eat and eat and eat and it will never satisfy you. You will feel sick before you feel satisfied," he explained. But by the end of a meal, you do—or at least should—feel reasonably sated. In that circumstance, you can eat something sweet and get pleasure from it, knowing that your feeling of fullness from the savory part of the meal should restrain you from gorging on sweets.

Although all infants have a sweet tooth, I had considerable help from my grandparents, Ben and Lena, who owned a grocery store offering a full line of candy. Not many people know my hometown—Kearny, New Jersey—or, if they do at all, it's as the location of the fictional Satriale's Pork Store in the title sequence of *The Sopranos.* My maternal grandparents had a small market in this old blue-collar town with black iron bridges and pre–World War II homes. I was a teenager before I conceded the fact that my grandma and grandpa owned a grocery store. To me it was a candy store. Even though the candy counter occupied 10 percent of the floor space, it held nearly all of my attention, except one time when I found a stack of "health magazines" featuring nude volleyball players, archers, and other athletes. They were captivating, but at the age of four I couldn't have told you why.

Onions, apples, coleslaw made fresh daily, bananas, salt, sugar, and potatoes left little impression on my memory. Instead, I recall Tootsie Roll Pops, Baby Ruths, baseball cards with big flat pieces of pink bubblegum coated in white powder so they wouldn't stick to the smiling photos of Mickey Mantle, Hank Bauer, and Whitey Ford. Also Tastykakes, Twinkies, Dugan's powdered donuts, Hershey bars, Nestlé Crunch, Good & Plenty, Necco Wafers, Bonomo's Turkish Taffy, Mike and Ike. A little later, about the time I became a Cub Scout, my horizons expanded to include Goldenberg Peanut Chews, Raisinets, and malted-milk balls that my mom and her girlfriends had at their weekly mah-jongg games.

Grandma and Grandpa also sold Breyer's ice cream, which was looked on with favor because it contained fresh fruit. Fresh anything was good in Grandma's book, including her all-purpose panacea and guarantor of good health, fresh air. Well into my twenties, I ate Breyer's ice cream on a daily basis. When I first moved to Brooklyn, there was a candy store in Flatbush that had blueberry Breyer's when blueberries were in season and peach ice cream during the peach harvest. Without putting it into words, because the term had not yet been invented, I felt a locavore emotion as I devoured those summer treats. In short, I love and have always loved sweets.

When I changed my diet, I didn't swear off sweets, I just curtailed them with surprising ease. It wasn't that hard to give up candy, but that still left me with the issue of dessert. Calvin Trillin deals with dessert by not ordering it. "I'm not a dessert guy," he told me. "I always thought if I craved dessert the way I craved a *banh mi* sandwich I'd weigh three hundred pounds. But I almost never order dessert in a restaurant. It's not that I don't like it, but I can sort of do without it."

I feel the same, but when I am in a restaurant where I am

known as a food writer, you can be sure that the chef will send out a flight—i.e., an assortment—of over-the-top desserts. I have learned to deal with this by not eating very much of any dessert while developing the art of rearranging things on the plate so that it always looks as if I have eaten more than in fact I have.

You have probably noticed that waiters often entreat customers to order dessert—in part, no doubt, because, as Daniel Boulud once told me, dessert can account for 15 percent of the profit on any check while incurring the minimal food costs of eggs, white flour, and white sugar. If there is no polite way around ordering dessert, my fallback is to order one for the table. This way, everyone gets a bite or two of a pacifying sugar fix.

Maintaining a healthy weight requires some form of truce with the practice of meal-ending sweets. Early in my food-writing career, I came up with the formulation "Never waste writing calories." By that I meant that I made it a practice to avoid foods that weren't really necessary.

Left to my druthers, like Trillin, I skip rich desserts, especially at home. This is much easier to do than kidding yourself that you are just going to have a bit of dessert. It is certain that one dish of ice cream in the third inning of a ball game will probably send you back to the freezer for a half-scoop an hour later, then a quarter-scoop for the seventh-inning stretch, and a final spoonful after turning off the TV.

My general rule of doing without dessert sometimes requires situational interpretation, as when someone has made something extra special because you are coming to dinner. Rather than appear like a spoilsport, I'll request a smaller piece of cake or pie and eat most but not all of it. However, when it is just my family in our home, and the urge strikes for something sweet to top off a meal, I will have fruit and a piece of dark chocolate.

Life is about choices. So is Culinary Intelligence. Look at it this way: a piece of apple pie has about as many calories as one and a half glasses of red wine; I choose the wine. To my mind, a meal without wine is a much less pleasurable prospect than a meal without, say, a chocolate volcano cake.

Sweet Beverages

Barry Popkin told me that for most of humankind's sojourn on this planet, we drank only two beverages: breast milk in infancy and then water. Nothing else. Every time you drink coffee or tea with milk, soda, juice, beer, wine, or hard liquor, you are adding significant calories to the original human diet. Furthermore, during the last half-century the world has gone on a soft-drink binge. We drink oceans of it. Small wonder that the obesity rate has gone up so dramatically.

Back when we were told that the only reason sodas were bad for you was that they caused cavities, every soft drink was sweetened with refined (white) cane sugar. I have my issues with refined sugar, but the soft-drink industry's current preferred sweetener, high-fructose corn syrup (HFCS), is even more of a dietary challenge. For all practical purposes, it is not chemically different from corn sugar, so it does no more harm. But since it is so cheap and is included in so many beverages (and other foods), it is, as Michael Pollan has persuasively pointed out, among the biggest contributors to the obesity epidemic. You might think that cutting out sodas will eliminate a lot of HFCS from your diet, but the same sweetener is used in sports drinks, even those endorsed by buff-bodied athletes.

Though some would argue that the added nutrients in sports drinks could conceivably do you some good, I doubt that they do very much, because they are isolated chemicals, not whole—or "real"—foods. The refined sugar and corn syrup in these beverages spike your production of insulin and add empty calories. During a recent hospitalization, my mom, when referring to the energy drink on her tray, would say, with undisguised irony, "Bring me a glass of Jonestown."

I am equally negative, or nearly so, when it comes to fruit juices. I am not anti-fruit. I love fruit. I eat a lot of it and have found it to be one of the best stavers-off of between-meal hunger pangs. Furthermore, fruits are loaded with all those vitamins that I don't get from the vitamin pills I don't take because every nutritionist I have spoken with has told me that a balanced diet that includes fruit and vegetables should have sufficient vitamins (well, okay, if you insist, maybe one multivitamin, which, like an atheist's death-bed prayer, can't hurt).

Fruit juice, even if it does contain vitamins, is nothing more than fruit with all the fiber removed, although juice with pulp left in does have fiber and is less rapidly absorbed. In other words, most juices are processed and refined down to two major ingredients, sugar and water. Seen purely in light of their effect on blood sugar, there isn't a whole lot of difference between apple juice, Wonder Bread, and an order of French fries. Fruits are whole foods. Fruit juices are processed.

As for artificially sweetened diet sodas and sports drinks, although they are not a caloric issue, I don't believe they do any good. They may help evade the guilt that comes with drinking sugary beverages, but a number of studies suggest that our taste receptors are not completely fooled by artificial sweeteners, so, paradoxically, they may in fact strengthen the urge to seek out sweetness in other foods. They deceive your taste receptors into thinking you are getting a sugar fix, but your body is not hoodwinked and the sweetness craving remains unsatisfied. Worse, these sweeteners are pure test-tube foods—the product of the laboratory rather than field, orchard, river, or ocean. They're the Partridge Family. For real satisfaction, what you want is the Rolling Stones.

Drinkies

"Hey, man, careful, there's a beverage here!"

—*The Big Lebowski*

Yes, alcoholic beverages are full of calories, but that alone is not an overriding reason to give up wine, beer, or the occasional cocktail. I haven't. These beloved libations have much to recommend them beyond their nutritional value. I always note with pleasure when research indicates that red wine might be heart-healthy, or that booze lowers stress levels, but I don't consume them as health supplements. As far as I am concerned, all I need to know is that alcohol in moderation is one of the pleasures that make eating a more complete and satisfying experience. Still, you can't escape the calories. There really is such a thing as a beer belly, to which you may add the notion of the wino waistline, the single-malt stomach, and the margarita midsection.

If you are seeking to control your weight, you have to monitor and, probably, moderate your drinking. This is one of those rules that young people don't think apply to them. I recall reading in the mid-1970s that Paul Newman drank a case of beer a day. He was thin and handsome, so I figured if I did what Paul Newman did it could only boost my studliness. I never got up to Newman's drinking level. In fact, on reflection, I'm not sure that he did either; perhaps his PR person took a six-pack or two of liberty with the truth. But, through perseverance and dedication, I often achieved a daily intake of three or four beers and two martinis. My body showed it.

I gave up my martini habit long before I attacked my weight problem. It happened when I discovered that my elder daughter, Lucy, who was three years old, was under the impression that the English-language word for "clear liquid in a glass" was "tini." From time to time, on special occasions, I will have one for old times' sake. Never two. In fact, now that I am out of the martini habit, two would put me under.

Even if you have the occasional cocktail, bear in mind that not all cocktails are created equal, at least when it comes to calories. Whereas a glass of scotch packs a caloric load, it doesn't measure up to drinks that include sugar *and* distilled liquor, such as Cosmopolitans, daiquiris, and Long Island Iced Teas. Adding sugar to alcohol in order to make the alcohol more palatable doesn't fit with any sensible weight-control strategy. Save such drinks, if at all, for very special occasions.

With all due respect, I'm assuming that if you drink alcoholic beverages you are a fibber when asked how much you throw back each day. This is not meant to pass moral judgment. I'm simply pointing out what I have observed to be a very consistent pattern of behavior among the drinking classes. Consider the following statement: "I usually drink about a glass of wine a day." If it were truly one glass and no more, you would not use the words "usually" and "about." It's a fair bet that you drink at least two glasses. If you said "a couple of glasses" (or, if asked the same question about beer, you answered "one or two"), I'm willing to wager that there are many days when "a couple" or "one or two" means at least three. No one overestimates their alcohol intake.

Set a limit and keep to it: one glass of wine or one beer at the beginning of your new regimen, and then two when you have reached your weight goal. For the most part, a cocktail equals two beers or two glasses of wine. When my status as a prediabetic encouraged me to reform my diet, I found that I could survive quite nicely with one glass (about five ounces) of wine with my main course. During this time, I was working in Argentina and Uruguay on a cookbook (*Seven Fires: Grilling the Argentine Way*). As you would expect, many of the recipes feature grilled meat. It was no surprise to find out that red wine—the kind of rich mouth-filling wine that goes so well with meat—is drunk in greater quantities there than anywhere else on earth.

The old me would have had three or four glasses. Instead, I started every meal with a glass of sparkling water, on the theory that, even though it is plain water and carbon dioxide, the bubbles do something interesting to your palate. When it came to the main event, the meat, I had a full glass of wine, and I savored it. Thinking about each sip surely contributed to enhancing the pleasure of the meal. Bottom line: at the end of the recipe-testing process, which extended over the course of that year, I had recaptured two inches of the most prized real estate, the notches on my belt.

High-Value Targets

It is certain that there are one or two high-calorie foods to which you are especially attached. It is no less certain that if you were to stop, or at least curtail, eating these things today, it would make a noticeable difference very soon. Often these are go-to foods that we have been eating so routinely for so long that we don't even think about them.

Among mine, pizza leads the list.

I have loved pizza since I first tasted it in July 1954 at the Pinebrook Auction, a North Jersey flea market cum tented bazaar. At my dad's suggestion, my mom ordered a slice of "pizza pie." No one simply said "pizza" back then; it was always "pizza pie." I was seven. I know that because that was the season the Yankees lost the pennant race to the Cleveland Indians. Prior to that, the Yankees had won five straight pennants and World Series, so I assumed that Yankees, pennants, and World Series wins were one and the same. Anyway, when my dad said "pie," it caught my attention. I liked pie. I watched with interest as my mom folded over a fresh slice and bit into it cautiously, so as not to burn her mouth.

"Hah," she said, which was as close as she could get to the word "hot" without burning her tongue on the bubbling mozzarella cheese and hot tomato sauce.

She offered me a taste. She blew on the slice to cool it down. At this point, my visual memory becomes a taste memory: sensual, nostalgic, and pleasant. Sweet, brightly acidic tomato, the hint of tooth resistance of the melted mozzarella, and the smooth, doughy mouth-feel of a well-charred crust that resolved in a crunch. It was spectacular!

From that day forward, I never thought that a slice of pizza wasn't a good idea. All through high school, my buddies and I would have pizza once, maybe twice a week. Two guys to an eight-slice pie, washed down with Coca-Cola poured over ice. We'd talk about girls, baseball, and cars—in that order.

These days, I am, for the most part, a stay-at-home writer, which means I sit down at my computer in the morning and keep working until I feel that I must have some lunch right away before I crash and pass out over my keyboard. Had I been more attentive to my body, I would have stopped before the need to eat felt like an emergency, but that's not the way I am.

So, pre-CI, when hunger would force me from my desk, I took advantage of the half-dozen good pizza shops within a few blocks of my house.

If you are a pizza lover, Brooklyn is as close to heaven as you are likely to get in this spin of the karmic wheel. Thicker or thinner, more or less char on the crust, fresh tomatoes or long-cooked sauce, garlic, basil, sausage imported from deepest Bensonhurst and Williamsburg. It is useless to kid yourself into thinking you are ever going to get away with just one slice.

"You're talking eight or nine hundred calories," my brother Donald the doctor said one day, when I'd explained my daily pizza routine to him.

Until Donald did the simple math, it had never occurred to me that tomatoes (a fresh whole food) and mozzarella (a freshly made cheese whose blandness leads one to think, incorrectly, that it is not high in calories) are not a light combination. It sure sounds Mediterranean and healthful. Let me clarify here that I am talking about New York pizza-shop pizza. I am not even considering the pizzas you see advertised on TV that have a very thick crust, which, in engineering terms, is required in order to support massive amounts of gooey cheese on top.

Sometime over the last twenty years or so, mass marketers have discovered that people think they are getting something extra special if their pizza is made with two, three, or four kinds of cheese. Most often, it's like mixing three wines in the same glass, to the detriment of each. Then there are the inevitable toppings—a usage that irks me. Not too long ago, toppings were things that you put on ice cream, like wet walnuts or chocolate sprinkles. But now toppings are part of the pizza lexicon. When we use a word that once connoted stuff that went on a hot-fudge sundae, it seems to me that we have crossed a conceptual line that encourages us to throw everything imaginable on a pizza.

Seen in this light, the modern mass-market pizza is more like a savory ice-cream sundae than nutritious food. Still, even the traditional simple pizzas served up by true pizza professionals are more likely to help put on weight than keep it off.

On the road to becoming slimmer, there was no choice but to cut out the daily pizza pilgrimage. The calculations worked out this way: if I was eating pizza five times a week, then a policy of pizza abstinence accounted for the caloric equivalent of one, or even two, whole days' worth of eating. Even the mathematically challenged (me) can see that you have a much better chance of losing weight when you don't try to cram nine days of eating into a seven-day week.

Your candidates for big calorie cuts may not match up with mine, but we are all creatures of habit, and I am sure you have some weight-boosting favorites: a croissant for breakfast, a chocolate-chip cookie reward after a salad-bar lunch, a scoop of butter-pecan ice cream during a *Seinfeld* rerun, or a couple of stiff drinks because it's Sunday.

My experience is not unique. I have seen cutting out White Stuff and picking off high-value targets (in my case pizza) work time and again. Kevin Stuessi is vice-president of the International Culinary Center (whose alumni include Dan Barber and Bobby Flay). He worked as a chef for Wolfgang Puck and Jeremiah Tower at Stars. He calls those two gigs "my moment of wow!" Later he opened the Bellagio for Steve Wynn in Las Vegas and then in Macau, China. In other words, the man was around a lot of food for a lot of years, and it showed. About two years ago, he gave up processed food and his own high-value target: not pizza, but a daily dose of ice cream. Long story short, he lost forty-five pounds in less than a year, and he has kept them off.

Cutting out just a few things from your habitual snack choices cannot help but save you thousands of calories. It is a sure way to get off on the right foot. But, then, there's always the metaphorical left foot, keeping the weight off. Your resolve is sure to weaken and ultimately fail unless you find your way to eating food that is more than merely healthy and just okay-tasting. If you are giving up some powerhouse tastes, you need to replace them with food that is equally satisfying, only much less full of things that declare war on your weight and your health.

Please note: I still have an occasional slice of pizza. Not once a day, not even once a week, but every now and again, because I still think there are few things that are more pleasurable to eat than pizza pie.

CHAPTER III It Starts with the Ingredients

"If you put good things in it, it will taste good," said the message on the business card of Caroline Rozgaj Kobe, a baker in Sugar Creek, Missouri. It was given to me by Kenny Yarnevic, a member of the Croatian Tailgaters at Arrowhead Stadium. You may come across longer and more labored explanations of nutritional theory; still, none do a better job of summing up half of the CI equation. Cooking is the other half, but ingredients come first.

I look at shopping for ingredients the way many NFL teams look at the college draft: pick the best from what is available. The only path to a truly healthful and enjoyable diet is to begin with great ingredients. Only by eating high-quality, well-prepared ingredients can you substitute satisfying and healthy food for the overly salty, fatty, sugary, highly processed, chemical-laden, crave-calming grub that accounts for so many of the items in any supermarket and on many restaurant menus. Flaccid tomatoes, mealy apples, limp greens, insipid pork, and tasteless beef cannot contribute to great flavor and texture. You can always resort to condiments and seasonings to rescue second-rate ingredients, but in the end you are left with the taste and calories of those extras, and little else.

In choosing ingredients, first consider plants. When planning a menu, chefs always do. We evolved to eat them, and they evolved to be eaten as a way of disbursing their seeds. We wouldn't eat them unless they tasted good, and they taste best when they carry the full complement of nutrients. Because they contain so much water by volume and their bulk is primarily fiber, a bite of fruit and vegetables will take up the same room in your stomach as a mouthful of steak, or banana-cream pie, but with far fewer calories.

Here we have another pillar of Culinary Intelligence: you can either fill up on high-calorie, high-fat, high-sugar food, or you can achieve the same degree of satiety from full-flavored ingredients. The key is "flavor." If it is not in the ingredient, you will seek it elsewhere—often to more fattening, less healthful effect. Eating fruits and vegetables because they are said to be "good for you" won't do the trick. Eating them because they taste good, will.

When chefs refer to a market-driven menu they are almost always talking about fruits and vegetables. Although the taste of grass-fed beef in June, spring lamb, summer salmon, or autumn pork may be superior, most animals that come to market are fed the same things all the time, so the natural seasonal variety in these ingredients is largely written out of the shopping equation. A good hunk of meat is a good hunk of meat.

Supermarkets may offer tomatoes, melons, and peaches year round, but the inescapable truth is that fruits and vegetables are only at their peak for a few weeks, or at most a month. If you buy out of season, you'll get better FPC from frozen or canned product harvested when ripe. We all know this, yet we continue to buy listless, puffy strawberries that are white on the inside and flavorless through and through, simply because the idea of strawberries on a bleak February day is appealing—if not for flavor, then at least for color.

Forget about it. The only thing blah strawberries can lead to is resorting to sugary syrup, calorie-rich whipped cream, or plain old sugar: in other words, attempting to salvage one inferior ingredient by adding other culprits is a surefire way to increase the useless-calorie count.

So—I wait to eat strawberries until June, when the local ones are dark red, about as large as a quarter, with a smell as sweet as a pot of jam. As for peaches, my favorite fruit, I admit to trying to jump the gun in July, when imports from South Carolina show up in the markets, and every so often I'll get a wonderful smooth, juicy-fleshed peach with psychedelic hints of honey and vanilla. But that's one peach out of a hundred. Even at their peak, in August in a good fruit year, I'd say the peaches at my local farmers' market are really great only 60 percent of the time, at best. If picked a few days too early, they are hard. If left to ripen in my pantry, by the time they are soft and sweet they are mushy in spots and borderline fermented in others. But when I strike peachy gold, a whole bag will serve for a few days' worth of workday snacks.

In August, the thought of a ripe peach always summons up memories of a lifetime of peach eating. Because food is one of the few experiences that can touch all of our senses, it lodges in memory through many pathways. For example, when I think of peaches I often recall coming into the breakfast room of an anglers' hotel in Esquel, Patagonia, the last stop on the old Patagonian Express, where I spent a few days fishing a beautiful meadow creek where pink flamingos gathered. The breakfast served in the little hotel couldn't have been simpler: coffee and, alongside the cup, a wooden board on which rested two fresh peaches, some Toblerone chocolate, and a stag-horn knife.

Such taste memories, and the scenes they evoke, are much more emotionally vivid than mere recall of facts or dates. Every time you eat a delicious fruit, you add that experience to the pleasure you will feel the next time you are served one. This in itself is an argument for the best ingredients: they make memory sweeter and the next experience that much richer. I have always supposed that Proust's immortal memory of a madeleine was reinforced by a lifetime's worth of madeleines dipped in tea.

In terms of savory produce, I take my cue from tomatoes. If a market, or a restaurant, offers great tomatoes, you have probably found yourself a place that also has bracingly fresh lettuce, basil with tender leaves and just a little licorice taste, or sweet peas that burst with the flavor of green growing things. If, on the other hand, an Italian restaurant serves *caprese* (salad of tomato, mozzarella, and basil) and the tomatoes are without flavor or texture, I would be willing to bet that the mozzarella is rubbery and the basil tough and bitter. The rest of the menu is probably not much better.

Too often, tomatoes in salads are put there for color, not for taste. They are harvested well before they are ripe on the vine. "There's no way that you can pack a tomato in California that rates two out of five on a color scale and have it taste like a five when it gets to New York," the West Coast buyer for one of the largest suppliers of organically grown tomatoes told me.

I recently went three whole years without tasting a great tomato. I couldn't chalk it up to the presumptive low quality of supermarket produce. In fact, I have noticed that increasingly more supermarkets sell some fresh local fruits and vegetables. Nor was the problem confined to the United States. Two visits to Italy, two to Spain, and three to Argentina and Uruguay—all of the trips food-related—featured similarly lackluster tomatoes, so it couldn't be blamed on a rainy New York summer, as happened in 2009.

"What gives?" I asked Carmine Cincotta, my friend and the owner of my local fruit and vegetable market, Jim & Andy's.

"They stopped growing old-time Jersey beefsteaks [or their equivalent on other continents], even in New Jersey. They're growing them with tougher skins now. I guess they don't lose as much from bruising in shipment," Carmine said disapprovingly.

Every shopper should have a Carmine in his or her life, but unless you live in an old big-city neighborhood, you may not. Fortunately, now that supermarkets have begun to include organic and, to some extent, local options, you may find someone at your market who is up-to-date about what's good and where it comes from. (If you speak Spanish, this may be an opportunity to put it to good use. I often wonder, where would our restaurants and food stores be without our growing Latino workforce?)

Carmine's family has been in the business for seventy years, which is precisely the span during which America went from a society made up of rural and urban communities to one where suburban sprawl pushed the farmscape to the hinterlands, away from everyday life.

We became customers at Jim & Andy's when our daughter Lucy was two years old. Melinda and I went shopping for something to serve to the parents at her party. We weren't overly worried about what to give the kids. In those days fruit juice, sliced apples, string cheese, and Pepperidge Farm Goldfish followed by the happy-birthday cake were the usual fare for young celebrants.

At that time Jim & Andy's supplied fruits and vegetables for the workday lunches of the cast and crew of *The Cosby Show* at Silvercup Studios in Queens. Among their favorites, according to Carmine, were baby vegetables served as crudités. Melinda thought they'd make perfect party food for our celebration: tiny pattypan squash, baby zucchini, sugar snap peas, little cauliflowers. We filled up two shopping bags with baby vegetables for our baby's party.

"Fifty-five dollars," Jim said as he rounded down the sum that he had quickly written out in pencil on the side of a brown paper bag. Jim always rounded down, never up.

"You deliver?" I asked.

"We do."

"Okay. Sixty-five Montague Street. Kaminsky. Name's on the buzzer."

"We don't deliver on that side of Atlantic Avenue."

"It's just a few blocks, and, hey, I just dropped fifty-five dollars on baby vegetables" (a considerable sum for those times and our bank account).

"You have a driver's license?" Jim asked.

"I do."

He tossed a set of car keys to me. "Blue Caddy. Across the street."

With that gesture, Jim won two new customers for life. You can see him peering out from his doorway between Gray Kunz and me on the back-flap photo of *The Elements of Taste.*

Jim & Andy's is one of the dwindling number of immigrant-Italian greengrocers that were once commonplace in many American cities. Their numbers were supplemented by Eastern European Jews (among them my maternal grandparents). From horse-drawn carts and storefronts, immigrants and their first- and second-generation offspring sold the bounty of local farms.

In the postwar era, as the sons and daughters of the early-twentieth-century wave of immigrant storekeepers migrated to the new suburbs, and out of the family businesses, another group of new arrivals moved into the retail vacuum left behind. The corner greengrocer became the corner mini-market, in many cases owned by Koreans who, despite a marvelous food culture, did not have longtime connections with local truck farmers. One could no longer find the ruby-red strawberries, the gnarly Jersey beefsteak tomatoes, the sweet white-kerneled ears of farm stand corn that my mom would always taste before buying within hours of their having been picked.

By the 1960s, supermarkets had come to dominate the food supply. The emphasis was on fast-growing produce, available all year round. Convenience and cost, not taste and nutrition, were the most important considerations, and seemed poised to wipe flavorful seasonal produce off the map. Organic food wasn't even an issue, except for crunchy, back-to-the-earth types.

In that same era, another countervailing factor began to reshape the American food world. Chefs such as Alice Waters in northern California, the late Jean-Louis Palladin of Washington, D.C., and André Soltner in New York City, dissatisfied with the ho-hum ingredients found in the markets, started to deal directly with farmers, offering a guaranteed outlet and a better price and/or a reliable customer for a superior product. This marked the beginning of a dining revolution that has spawned thousands of farm-to-table restaurants and attracted ever-growing numbers of customers who delighted in great food prepared by gifted chefs.

But a relative handful of pioneering chefs would not have had much effect on our enormous country if the same kind of people who formed the clientele of the new American restaurants had not displayed an equal interest in preparing great food at home—as evidenced by the popularity of Julia Child's television show and, later, the *Silver Palate* cookbooks. Like the chefs at their favorite restaurants, enthusiastic home cooks sought better ingredients. Small farmers, who had survived the paving of America and the consolidation of its food supply, suddenly had a new marketplace.

Out of these converging circumstances, the contemporary greenmarket-and-farmers'-market movement was born. Today, you'll find farmers' markets in Los Angeles, New York, and San Francisco, as you would expect, but I have also sampled the produce in great farmers' markets in New Orleans, Bozeman, Des Moines—in fact, wherever I travel in America. There are more than seven thousand farmers' markets in the nation: a drop in the bucket compared with the number of supermarkets, but in terms of fostering a connection to really good, wholesome produce, they have been, to borrow a term from the book of Isaiah, a saving remnant.

Conventional retailers, rather than cede new business to small independent producers, began to move into this market segment with the birth of such supermarkets as Whole Foods, Fairway, Wegmans, Zingerman's, Bi-Rite, Corti Brothers, Hen House Markets, and Dorothy Lane, to name a few. Now even everyday nonpremium supermarkets often have local and organic sections, but it's not yet time to declare victory in the war to reclaim the flavor that was once the great gift of our farms and orchards. Informed consumers, who know good from bad, and are willing to pay a bit more for the good stuff, are necessary.

By the simple act of making a purchase of local ingredients you are voting with your pocketbook for sustainable, often organic produce. If you feel a little more moral for doing it, you are entitled. But feeling socially and environmentally responsible in your food shopping doesn't speak directly to the quality of the ingredients.

"It's not enough, you need to shop intelligently," Russ Parsons, the food editor of the *Los Angeles Times,* told me. Russ has written extensively and well about farmers, farming, and the pursuit of great ingredients. On a trip to the West Coast, Melinda and I met him for lunch at the Lazy Ox Canteen, a gastropub in Little Tokyo, a few blocks from the newspaper. We started with brick-roasted mussels in a chili sauce. As I write this sentence, I realize I had no idea what "brick-roasted" meant, but it sounded so honest and straightforward that I was sold. Another starter, beef-tongue ravioli stuffed with creamy yogurt and pine nuts, made me reconsider the unflattering things I have said about this insufficiently esteemed cut of meat. Similarly, the lowly skate—which most fishermen I know discard as trash—was served up on an intensely flavorful corn-and-stewed-tomato pudding. The green salad was simple, sublime, and fresh.

"These greens are insane," I said to the waiter. "Farmers' market?"

"Nope. Sage Mountain Farm, about eighty miles southeast of L.A."

They had been bought direct from the farmer, not from the greenmarket we had passed on our walk to lunch, where the produce on that day, at least, did not fairly shout with freshness and peak flavor. I asked Russ if his experience with farmers' markets in recent years had been the same as mine: some great stuff, much more average stuff, and even a little forgettable stuff.

"Definitely," he said. "The thing about shopping at farmers' markets is, many people don't really shop. They show up and then fill their bags at the first stand they hit. I like to walk around the market, see what looks good, try a few things, feel others. It's not all the same." With that comment, Russ had put his finger on the pitfall of going to the greenmarket and leaving your food sense at home. There will still be good and not-so-good from which to choose.

In other words, greenmarket shopping is no different from any other kind of shopping. For instance, if you go to buy shoes, don't you try them on first? Apply this same principle to buying fruits and vegetables. Touch them gently. Do they feel like living—or recently living—things? Are they granite-hard or soft as cornmeal mush? If vendors object to touching, and don't offer samples, I spend my money elsewhere.

Before you buy a cantaloupe—or anything else, for that matter—smell it. That's the primary reason you have a nose: to lead you toward good food and away from not-good food. If a fruit or vegetable has beautiful aroma, you can start to feel right about buying it. Definitely ask for a taste. Most greenmarket folks will be glad to oblige you. The enterprising ones probably already have some of their best produce cut up and ready to sample. If they don't, then for things like apples or pears, worst case, you drop fifty cents and buy one to try. That's better than spending six dollars for a bagful that can only be salvaged as applesauce or puréed pears.

In my region, the ripeness of produce usually progresses south to north and from lowlands to hill country. If I see blueberries in July or peaches in early August, I know that in most years the first really great local ones will be from South Jersey, or Pennsylvania. And if this is the case, I know that by the following week or so the Central and North Jersey farmers will have peaches at their peak, followed by New York State growers in the following week. After that, I'll probably have to look for produce from farther north, but that will bump up against the limit of the fresh-fruit-and-vegetable foodshed.

This is not to suggest that there is an official border between one foodshed and another. It's more of a rule of thumb that, the farther a fruit or vegetable has to travel, the earlier it must be picked and the less flavor and pleasing texture it will have developed. Practically speaking, the limit of a foodshed is the distance that a farmer can drive in one day, tend to a stand in the market, and return that evening. This would put the boundary of peak flavor at approximately 150 miles.

Fruits develop full sweet flavor and great texture only when they are mature and ready to drop off the tree, bush, or vine. Many vegetables, on the other hand, can be harvested when they are still immature. Their flavor is quite good and the texture is delightful, even superior. These baby vegetables are more expensive per pound, which makes sense. Had the farmer left the lettuce or carrot or eggplant to mature, it would have weighed more, probably fetching a higher price. Baby or grown-up, what matters most is how carefully the vegetables have been raised, the soil, and the climate in which they grow.

After they are harvested, the issue is not simply food miles per se but how fruits and vegetables are cared for while in transit, and how long they have been out of the ground, off the branch, or off the vine. One immutable law is that the longer the interval between harvest and plate, the greater the loss of flavor and texture.

One can't discuss local markets without mentioning locavores, i.e., people who eat locally sourced food. Nice concept, ugly word. There are many reasons why eating local makes good sense. The concepts of food miles and mindfulness of the energy costs of transporting and storing food are valid from both an economic and environmental point of view. But these are quite separate considerations from how the food tastes. Often local origin goes hand in hand with flavor and taste, but not always. The farmer still needs to grow and gather with care.

"But what do you eat in January?" is the most common challenge leveled at the locavore. The first part of my answer is purely practical; I am a locavore when there is local to be had. There is a particular pleasure in eating with the seasons. Just as baseball gives way to football, and football gives way to March Madness, I find myself anticipating the first peas of spring, the strawberries of June, the peaches and tomatoes of August, the apples and butternut squash of autumn. I root for them as enthusiastically as I cheer on my team. As a sports fan, I want my local teams to win. With fruits and vegetables, great flavor constitutes a win.

Part two of my answer is equally nondogmatic: you do what you can. Please note: fruits and vegetables include more than peaches, corn, and tomatoes. Well after the harvest moon, brussels sprouts, cabbage, pumpkins, apples, pears, turnips, carrots, parsnips, chard, kale, cauliflower, beets, onions, and leeks are all available.

This late-season list may not inspire you the way summer produce does. Perhaps the simple explanation is that winter produce lacks the bright colors of summer. For months on end, though, I am happy to use autumn and winter produce to make great soups, sautéed greens, oven-roasted root vegetables. Dried herbs, bacon or salt pork, raisins, black olives, pine nuts, pepper flakes, and garlic liven up and add depth of flavor to most of these ingredients, as will letting them cook in the pan juices alongside a roast. Beans, lentils, and chickpeas, fortified with stock and wine, make warming and restorative winter meals. A side salad of shaved raw Brussels sprouts dressed in olive oil and lemon juice, seasoned with salt and tossed with crumbled feta cheese, is as fresh-tasting, if not quite as delicate, as August greens (see page 239).

Good as late-season ingredients can be, it's also true that in the depths of February I will gladly eat good trucked-in or flown-in product. It seems foolish to completely reject our sophisticated global freight network. Remember, the objective of CI is flavor and quality, not just localness. So Arizona greens, Central American bananas, HoneyBell oranges from Florida, pink grapefruit from Texas, California cherry tomatoes, all find their way into my winter cooking. No doubt they are better tasting when picked ripe and served close to home, but when you need a fresh-fruit fix in the worst midwinter way, they do the trick.

At that same time of year, I don't dismiss all out-of-season greenhouse produce as tasteless artifacts of the food-industrial complex. Under the right conditions, greenhouse fruits and vegetables can be terrific, not just a source of seasonally disoriented plants.

Dan Barber is an eloquent and accomplished writer on the subject of sustainability, and the chef and proprietor of Blue Hill at Stone Barns, a farm cum restaurant on the site of the former dairy of David Rockefeller and his wife, Peggy. In addition to fields and gardens on the picturesque and bucolic property, there are huge greenhouses, nearly twenty-five thousand square feet, where Dan and his colleagues raise vegetables all year. If you visit him in mid-January, a salad of baby greens and fresh herbs arrives at your table as pleasingly as a January thaw.

On one late winter's day, he invited me up to discuss raising hogs on pasture, a feeding regime that I had written about in my book *Pig Perfect: Encounters with Remarkable Swine.*

I followed him to the greenhouse. We walked into the sweet, wet smell of a garden and recently turned topsoil. Barber, in chef's tunic and white apron, dug a carrot out of the ground. Black soil, the product of Stone Barns' prodigious compost heaps, clung to a carrot that almost glowed orange.

I thought of an old Irish folk saying that I learned from Sean Kelly, one of my colleagues at *National Lampoon.* "You have to eat a peck of dirt before you die," his grandmother would tell him whenever the youngsters got picky with the food that was placed in front of them. This left young Sean—who had a Jesuitical cast of mind—unclear on which was the preferable course: eating dirt or avoiding it. The sense of Grandma Kelly's advice, no doubt, was that we shouldn't worry about a little dirt on our food because everyone ends up eating at least a peck of it during the course of a lifetime. But Sean, whose hairsplitting drove the brothers in catechism class to consider an exorcism, wondered, "Well, if I have to eat a peck before I die, does that mean I should worry that every bit of dirt will bring me closer to the grave?"

Dan had no such concerns. After dusting the soil off with a few flicks of a kitchen towel that he wore on his shoulder, he snapped the freshly dug carrot in two, and we tasted: very intense, really sweet.

"The sugar level is off the charts," he said. "And it's not just sugary. It's like wine."

"Something else, Dan," I said, detecting a surprising nuance in the flavor: like marzipan.

"Almonds," Dan said. "I've been putting ground-up almond shells in the carrot beds. It's a trick I picked up from the French guy who sells me these crazy-expensive but fabulous oils pressed from almonds, pistachios, and walnuts."

Seasoning the soil. It made sense.

When I reminded him of this conversation a few years later, Dan wrote back that he had developed this line of thought even further than his small-scale greenhouse-carrot experiment, and taken it into his outdoor garden. "You can write a kind of recipe for, say, a carrot, long before it gets to your kitchen. I believe that this attention to a recipe from the ground up is going to be the future of being a chef. If you get the soil right, it's possible to pre-salt, pre-sweeten, and eliminate (sort of) the need for extra fat, because one of fat's main roles is to carry flavor." Or, to put it another way, he is putting CI in the soil. I really like this idea.

These days, any serious discussion of fruits and vegetables is incomplete without a consideration of organic versus nonorganic produce. Common sense suggests that keeping chemical fertilizers out of the soil, chemical sprays off of our vegetables, and antibiotics out of our livestock is desirable. It certainly is important to the long-run health of Mother Earth.

Still, just because a fruit or vegetable is organic doesn't guarantee that it will be great-tasting, although it often is. Other things being equal, I will always opt for produce grown according to organic practices, especially when I have had a good experience with the merchant or grower. This is not always the same as "certified organic," a bureaucratically defined status whose achievement besets farmers with requirements that are sometimes not practical for the small-scale producer. Organic certification can be a good thing, but the best guide is to know your producers or buy from someone who does and whom you trust.

And so we come to the last line of defense that the subsidy-driven processed-food system puts up against seasonal, local, full-flavored ingredients—the charge of elitism.

"You can afford them," I often hear, "but what about the average person?" I find this concern for the common man unconvincing, especially when advanced by the PR arm of a big corporation.

Furthermore, when local produce is in season, this accusation is factually untrue. I have never come across a better counter to this argument than the one offered by Jonathan Waxman, the Vegas trombone player turned super-chef at Chez Panisse and eventually at a string of Manhattan restaurants beginning with the storied Jams, one of New York's first modern fine-dining restaurants. "Here's my philosophy," Waxman said. "You have a farmers' market where things are in season, and you buy things when they're in season because they're more plentiful. When you buy peas or asparagus when they're in season, they're cheap. When you buy them out of season, or from a faraway place, that's when they're expensive. That's how the markets work."

The question is not one of food aristocrat versus commoner. It's really, where do you choose to spend your money? I would rather risk being thought a healthy elitist than risk becoming a dangerously overweight populist. But that answer, like the accusation of elitism, is too simplistic.

Think of it this way. A turnip on sale at a local greenmarket is made up of one ingredient—itself—and nothing by way of expensive packaging, labeling, or additives. On the other hand, processed vegetables like, for example, the beloved Tater Tots of my earlier years, are dosed with chemical additives that are devised at substantial cost to large corporations, in the form of the work of university-trained chemists with expensive postgraduate degrees. They (the Tater Tots, not the chemists) are sealed in packages created by engineers on an assembly line designed by still other expensively pedigreed engineers. The packages are made to look appealing by skilled artists and designers. The finishing verbal touches on the package are put there by clever writers adept at making nonactionable health claims and seductive taste promises, often on the instruction of psychologists who have focus-grouped the names of the products and the attributes that the public finds attractive—never mentioning that the chemicals, calories, heavy salting, and saturated fats in their product cannot contribute to a balanced and wholesome diet. Throw in vetting by lawyers whose hourly rates look like a ZIP code.

In other words, in distinction to the unadorned turnip and the farmer who plants and harvests this humble root, the Tater Tot team marshals a platoon of PhD scientists and many dollars in consumer research, industrial engineering, expensive transportation, and storage, while the big growers that supply the potatoes reap large tax subsidies. Seen in this light, choosing simple, mostly seasonal, mostly local ingredients rather than processed products doesn't seem quite so elitist as the assumption that corporate alchemy will create better foods than those that nature gives us.

Meatland

Chefs, food writers, and Death Row prisoners are often asked what they would like for their last meal. In the case of chefs and food writers, this question is presumably posed as a "What if?," but for condemned murderers it's a bona-fide request for a dinner order. One theme runs through all the responses: nobody contemplates saying goodbye to this life with a plate of vegetables. In the United States, steak leads the prisoners' list, although burgers, fried chicken, and pork chops make frequent appearances—sometimes all together, as they did when Bobby Wayne Woods put in the following order: "Two fried chicken breasts; three fried pork chops; two hamburgers with lettuce, tomato, onion, and salad dressing; four slices of bread; half a pound of fried potatoes with onion; half a pound of onion rings with ketchup; half a pan of chocolate cake with icing; and two pitchers of milk." Not exactly a healthy diet, but, then, Bobby Wayne wasn't thinking long-term.

The truth communicated by these farewell feedings is that human beings love meat. We have been eating it for as long as we have been human, probably longer. In terms of nutrient density it is nonpareil. You would think, then, that diet gurus would universally embrace meat eating, and that their millions of followers would do the same. However, because consuming meat is so intricately bound up with the question of life and death, it is fraught with emotional and ethical overtones.

I do not doubt that the concern of vegetarians for animals is genuine. I too am distressed when animals are abused and degraded to provide us with cheap meals. I wrote a whole book about the pork industry and its shortcomings, both moral and nutritional. With the help of two farmers and one professor in the Carolinas, I bought and raised two dozen free-ranging, acorn-eating pigs. They lived a better and longer life than their factory-farm counterparts. They were absolutely delicious, too.

Meat eating is held by some to be a barbaric holdover from humanity's childhood. This position does not adequately take into account the fact that at some point *everything* that lives gets eaten, or, according to an Argentine folk saying: *"Todo bicho que camina va a parar al asador"* (loose translation: "Sooner or later, every critter ends up on the grill"). So it's just a question of whether you eat that steak, or the scavengers, worms, and microbes do. Some organism is going to digest it.

This truth hit home for me quite forcefully about ten years ago, when an assignment took me to the Serengeti, in Tanzania. A herd of elephants had left unmistakable signs of their passage. I still have a photo of myself holding a piece of elephant dung, about the size of a softball, which I sent to my chef friends. "*Prior to marinating*," I wrote. Bear in mind that elephants eat enormous quantities of leaves and twigs, most of it indigestible, so their dung is like a clump of straw. At my feet, where more elephant droppings lay, a column of beetles stretched across the road, each of them carrying a mini-load of elephant poo.

Farther on down the road I picked up the skull of a wildebeest, every trace of flesh licked clean by scavengers, insects, microbes. What was left of the bones looked more like a honeycomb than a smooth white surface, because still other tiny creatures had sucked every minuscule morsel of nutrition from the bone structure, leaving only skeletal remains to bleach in the sun and ultimately return their minerals to the soil.

We turned off the road and came upon a pride of lions devouring a freshly killed wildebeest. The lions departed, wanting no part of us or our Land Rover, which I think they regarded as a larger, competing carnivore. A lone vulture descended and began to peck at the wildebeest innards. Soon the ravenous bird was joined by two dozen of his fellow carrion eaters. Their heads were smeared with blood as they ripped at the wildebeest carcass, but, apart from the gore, I couldn't shake the impression that they looked like a group of bald old men.

At that moment, I first fully realized—perhaps because I was witnessing it for myself rather than watching it on the National

Geo Channel—that every fleet-footed plant eater (zebra, wildebeest, impala) has a predator (lion, leopard, cheetah) that, under the right conditions, can overtake its prey. Likewise, for every predator there are scavengers that feast on its flesh when its day comes, and so on through the great chain of being, until every animal and every plant returns to the earth to be recycled as nutrients for coming generations of living things. It's unclear in this scenario why our forswearing meat eating will improve nature's balance.

That we evolved to consume meat is scientifically indisputable. There is no way our species would have developed functionally different teeth to cut meat, shear vegetables, and grind nuts and grains if we hadn't evolved to eat an omnivore's diet. Nature doesn't waste her time perfecting useless DNA. Humans are meant to eat meat.

We weren't, however, designed to eat bad meat. By "bad" I don't mean tainted or spoiled, I mean bland, almost tasteless meat that is obtained from animals raised in brutal confinement pens, pumped up with hormones and antibiotics, fed crops grown on land where the rain forest has been clear-cut to enable the production of genetically modified corn and soy that is grown with the use of petroleum-based fertilizers. Such meat is harmful to the health of those who consume it, and its production takes a great toll on our world.

But a free-range steer, or a lamb raised on salty grass by the sea, or a pig allowed to roam oaken forests—these are incomparable treats and have an important place in the scheme of Culinary Intelligence. Eating good meat, although it is often more expensive than industrially produced meat, contributes to a varied diet, so the price of Monday's costly cut of veal is offset—usually more than offset—by Tuesday's mushroom risotto and Wednesday's pasta. More flavorful meat, because of its superior sensorial qualities, is more satisfying. You can eat less and enjoy more. On this subject of sensual satisfaction, Thomas Keller wrote in his comprehensive service manual for the French Laundry:

> All menus at the French Laundry revolve around the law of diminishing returns such as the more you have of something the less you enjoy it. Most chefs try to satisfy a customer's hunger in a shorter time with one or two main dishes. The initial bite is great. The second bite is fabulous. But on the third bite, the flavors lessen and begin to die. The fabulous first impression is lost and the diner soon loses interest.

He formulated these instructions by way of explaining his multi-hour, multi-course meals. My goal as an eater, and as a cook, is to get a similarly high degree of satisfaction out of whatever I eat. To be sure, in a normal home-cooked meal of a main course and a couple of side dishes, I don't expect to be satisfied with Keller's three bites, but two or three slices of a great rib eye is all I need as an entrée. If the ingredients are good and prepared well, with a flavorful crust and fully developed meaty flavor, there should never be a need to go back for seconds and thirds. When you do, I think you are probably motivated not so much by hunger as by lack of satisfaction, because flavor is missing.

And if meat doesn't have flavor, then a typical recourse is to smother it in sauce, usually high in calories, salt, fat, and, often, sugar. For example, consider conventional corn-fed filet mignon, a costly cut of beef. What it has to recommend it is that it looks nice and is exceedingly tender. What it doesn't have is deep flavor, which is why béarnaise sauce, compound butters, and other flavor boosters are often pressed into service. I observed the merits and shortcomings of grain-fed filet mignon when Lucia Soria, a talented Argentine chef, came to New York to help test recipes for the *Seven Fires* cookbook. I wanted to make sure the recipes worked in the U.S.A. with our ingredients and hardwoods.

Argentine beef is free-ranged on grass. It has deep, wild flavor. So, for our daylong cookout in my backyard, I bought grass-fed cuts for much of the testing, but grass-fed filet mignon is just about impossible to find. Why? Because grass-fed animals tend to be leaner: they lack the marbling that makes meat tender. Thus, the tenderloin of a grass-fed steer is tougher than its grain-fattened counterpart. That's why most Argentines' steak of choice is the rib eye, which is shot through with the intramuscular fat that is the hallmark of a mature, well-exercised free-range animal.

I was able to find grass-fed rib eyes, strip steaks, and rib roasts at Staubitz Market and Paisano Brothers (my local butchers), but as for the other cuts: *nada.* This didn't matter too much with cross-cut short ribs (*costillas* in Spanish, or *flanken* in Yiddish), which are a traditional starter course at an Argentine cookout. They are chewy and crusty—whether grass- or grain-fed.

Among the recipes we tested was filet mignon wrapped in fresh sage leaves and bacon. When we made this in South America with grass-fed beef, it had immense flavor—the floral, herbal sage, the smoky, salty, porky bacon, and, most of all, the funky and umami tastes of a grass-fed animal.

However, when we made the same recipe in my backyard in Brooklyn, Lucia tried a piece fresh off the grill and said, "I taste the sage and the bacon, but the meat has absolutely no flavor."

To be fair, it had some flavor, but certainly not enough to stand up to sage and bacon. In nature, cattle exercise their muscles and eat grass: it's what suits them and gives them flavor. They don't naturally eat corn. Nothing naturally eats corn, because corn doesn't exist in a wild form in nature. It is completely a hybrid, the result of human ingenuity.

This all happened about ten thousand years ago, before humans domesticated grain in the Old World. Native American farmers in present-day Mexico succeeded in interbreeding three ancestral grasses that grew hundreds of miles apart. This means, not only were these people accomplished agronomists, but they carried out trade over long distances. I admire them for it. I like corn and I eat it. But it does not change the fact that cattle evolved to eat grass, which packages its nutrients in much less gigantic grains. I prefer the taste of grass-fed beef, even though it does not have the same amount of tenderizing marbling as a corn-fattened animal.

Corn-fed or grass-fed, though, if meat doesn't start out with intrinsic flavor that can be developed through kitchen skill, then meat eaters will turn to flavor enhancers to intensify the experience. The meat itself becomes an afterthought: it's no more than a platform that adds texture but little in the way of flavor.

Most supermarket pork is an example of taste-deficient meat. More than 90 percent of America's pork comes from pigs raised in confinement in horrific factory farms. Compared with the deep, rich, juicy flavor of Spanish pigs that forage for acorns (the preferred food of all pigs in the wild), such commodity pork is bland, tasteless, and dry. There is no way to make a flavorful silk purse, so to speak, out of an industrially raised sow's ear, so we pour on the sugary, cornstarch-thickened, chemically laden barbecue sauces in an attempt to achieve some of the pleasure that industrialized meat can never offer.

If you doubt this, you might make a pilgrimage to the Lourdes of barbecuing, the Memphis in May Festival, on the banks of the Mississippi River at that bewitching time of year when spring in the South is poised to burst into full summer. Wreathed in the meat-perfumed smoke of hundreds of cooking fires, the festival site sprawls along the grassy riverside just downstream of the

Memphis-Arkansas Bridge. Still swollen with spring's flood, the muddy torrent carries branches ripped from trees a thousand miles upstream and sweeps them to the Gulf of Mexico.

Lining the shore you will find ranks of huge, gaily decorated, smoke-belching, very expensive barbecue rigs belonging to the competing pit masters. Beside each rig, a fancifully appointed tented area offers shade as well as shelter from the thunderstorms that boil out of the hot, humid heartland. The scene looks and feels like a midway at an old-time county fair. "Pork Me Tender," proclaimed one Elvis-themed tent when I visited; "The Pork Authority," declared another, beneath a replica of the Statue of Liberty. And then there was this head scratcher, which left me wondering if a branch of the Kaminsky clan of Narev, Poland, might have found their way to the West Indies: "Herb's Jamaican Style Polish Sausage."

There were grand masters representing all the denominations of the pork-barbecue faith: whole hog, spareribs, sausages, shoulders. Some were better than others, but all quite good and all potently flavored, after they had been seasoned, long-smoked, injected with peach or apple juice, dusted with secret formulae of onion powder, celery salt, garlic, ginger, black pepper, cayenne, white pepper, paprika, and even more super-double-secret sauces of ketchup, mustard, vinegar, sugar, maple syrup, and more cayenne.

"But," I wondered, "how does the pork itself really taste?"—which seemed, after all, to be the original point of the exercise. Had this escaped the tens of thousands of people who lined up eagerly to scarf down their 'cue?

Don't get me wrong: what I ate in Memphis was delicious, as you would expect when you let the combination of pork, heat, smoke, salt, and time work its sorcery. But if you're looking for the natural taste of pork, you probably won't get much at any barbecue competition. When I smoke shoulders or ribs, I brine them, season them with salt and smoky hot paprika, and leave them in the smoker for a good long while at about 220 degrees. If I dress my meat at all, a splash of vinegar and some red pepper flakes for pulled shoulder is the sum total. The flavor of the pork comes through in a subtly seductive way that no amount of barbecue sauce can equal, and which, in fact, it often obscures.

My vote is to skip the bottled sauces. Enjoy the pork fully. In fact, the best piece of pork I ever tasted was seasoned with salt—and nothing more—and thrown into a hot pan. In my two-year search for the greatest ham in the world, I stopped in the little village of Aracena, in the west of Spain. I had traveled there because that region is the home turf of the *pata negra* (black-foot pig) and the exquisite *jamón ibérico,* made from free-range, acorn-fattened, super-succulent swine. Tipping the scales at 350 pounds (compared with American hogs, usually slaughtered at about 180 pounds), these animals are loaded with monounsaturated (i.e., heart-healthy) fat, just like olive oil. The current marketing mantra of the consortium of ham makers rhapsodizes about the *ibérico* hog as "the four-footed olive tree."

Bar Manzano sits just off the main square of Aracena, one of the "white villages" of Spain—so called because of the color of the buildings that the Moors erected when they ruled here a thousand years ago. On a cold winter's night, with snow on the mountaintops, and a full moon lighting the ruins of the medieval fortress that overlooks the town, the world takes on the day-for-night silver sheen of a black-and-white movie.

As in almost every restaurant in Spain, the bar at Bar Manzano holds an array of olives, sausages, roasted Marcona almonds, and a big *torta española*—kind of a quiche with potatoes that are precooked in olive oil. Serving as a backdrop to the *torta,* the handles of draft-beer spouts invite the new arrival to slake his thirst. A cold beer is not the first thing that comes to mind on such a night, but since all the locals were drinking beer, the foam dripping off their mustaches, I went with the custom and ordered one. I love Spanish beer. Its crisp sharpness cuts through the prevailing saltiness of tapas.

My ham cicerone, Miguel Ullibari, introduced me to the chef/owner, Susi Del Prado, a lovely young woman who invited me into her kitchen.

"Do you know about the secret?" she asked, in Spanish.

"Secret?" I echoed.

Grabbing a thin slice of pork, she plunked it down on the counter and said, "This—they call it the secret—it comes from just beneath the diaphragm. On a big pig, a hundred fifty kilos, there's only one little piece like this, and it weighs less than a kilo, but it is the best."

As she spoke, she placed a skillet on the flame, salted the meat, and tossed it in the pan. No oil. This surprised me, but then, in a matter of seconds, fat—deliciously nutty-smelling—began to weep out of the pork. She continued to cook it until it developed a gorgeous crust. She slipped it onto a plate. I cut off a piece with my pocketknife. The flavor was marvelously full, rich, and savory, with deep umami, and nothing more had been done to it than transforming it through heat and seasoning. If I ever needed proof that the quality of the prime ingredient is the most important thing in cooking, this *secreto* proved it. Even with a sauce that she made with whiskey, olive oil, bay, and garlic, the pork came through as the fundamental flavor. It was as delicious and pure in its way as a glass of Burgundy, a slice of summer cantaloupe, a fried egg with salt and black pepper.

To find good-tasting meat, you need to seek it out. If you live in a neighborhood with a butcher, get acquainted. Ask questions. Make requests. Having a relationship—especially if you are spending cash—is the best way I know to find a source of quality meat. It is no longer so easy as it was when every town and every neighborhood had a local butcher.

Years ago, before it had gone from being marginally sketchy to entry-level gentrified, I lived in Park Slope, Brooklyn. The local Realtors touted it as "the largest Victorian-era neighborhood in America." Think Sesame Street with no puppets.

On Sunday mornings, I would walk across Prospect Park and then through Kensington—a working-class neighborhood with clapboard houses from the 1920s. Because it was sheltered from the winds off the harbor and received a lot of sunlight, it was the first place in my immediate world where crocuses bloomed in the spring. After a New York winter, the sight of those tiny flowers was like a postcard from an old friend.

My destination was Church Avenue in Borough Park. Whenever I took that two-mile hike, I would get a brisket from Saul Taub, who was, as his sign proclaimed in both English and Hebrew, a kosher butcher.

Morning light often poured through his window. When it did, it was a good bet you would find Saul's well-fed cat basking in the sunlight, licking his sleek and shiny coat. Being a butcher's cat is a good gig.

I'd always enter to the same scene. Sawdust on the floor. On the radio, the races from Aqueduct, called in Yiddish. Three or four wooden folding chairs usually occupied by a lineup of old ladies, pocketbooks on their laps, intent on Saul's technique. I'd watch too. If, while he was grinding an order of chopped meat, some of the fat that he used to push the meat through the grinder happened to emerge in long squiggles, the lady who had placed the order would leap out of her chair like a rocketing pheasant and berate Saul for sneaking in some cheap fat in place of costly meat.

With an uncombative sigh and a slight smile, he'd always give the same answer to the glowering grandmas: "Don't worry, I wouldn't charge extra."

After I'd been his customer for five or six years, he told me the story behind the number tattooed on his wrist.

"I was a boy, thirteen years old. The Nazis put me in a concentration camp. It was late in the war. One day, we all knew the Russians were approaching the camp. You could hear their cannons. The Germans took us all outside, made us strip, and began shooting.

"When I heard the first shot, I fell. I pretended I was hit. The bodies piled up on top of me. Then the shooting stopped. I lay there for hours. Quiet. The Russian guns grew louder. Finally, I heard soldiers speaking Russian, so I climbed out through the pile of dead bodies.

"It was very cold. A young Russian took off his heavy wool overcoat and gave it to me. I walked three hundred miles back to Czechoslovakia."

After ten years of Saul's briskets and kosher chickens, I moved to L.A. for a few years. When I returned to New York, my brother Don and I made the long walk to Saul's for old times' sake. Same cats. Same ladies. Same frantic announcer on the radio screaming, "*Er loift vie Secretariat!*" ("He runs like Secretariat!").

Saul touched the tip of his cap. It was his way of saying hello.

We sat in the empty chairs at the end of the queue and worked our way forward. When it came my turn, Saul, who hadn't seen me in two years, went into the meat locker and emerged with a brisket.

"You want I should trim the fat?" he asked.

Butchers like Saul are mostly a thing of the past. Finding good-tasting meat, sustainably raised (sustainability was not on the radar in my Saul Taub years), requires a bit of research, usually on the Internet. Try the key phrase "heritage breeds" in your ZIP code. Although most supermarket meat is factory-farmed, or at least raised on a regimen of antibiotics and growth hormones, good-tasting meat from sustainable producers is increasingly more available even in supermarkets. Ask for the manager of the meat department. Be open to his or her suggestions. You'll be surprised how many of these "anonymous" employees respond to a personal approach.

There are branded producers who have begun to fill the need for good-quality meat. I trust the Niman Ranch brand. The Berkshire Gold pork program delivers a quality product. Heritage Foods USA ships wonderful meats to consumers. Companies like Fresh Direct deliver to your door. The list of quality brands is growing. Here and there around America, restaurateurs who have built up a clientele with a taste for great meat have begun to open artisanal butcher shops. Your farmers' market is also an option. So is joining a co-op or CSA (Community Supported Agriculture). Things are getting better for carnivores if they do their homework.

Shopping for great meat is no different from shopping for great produce. Five words should guide you:

Look,
Ask,
Cook,
Taste,
Learn.

Seafood: A Tale of Two Shrimp

Try this experiment. Take some defrosted shrimp out of the fridge.

"But," you say, "these shrimp that I just bought for $12.99 a pound weren't frozen to begin with."

Yes, they were, or at least I am pretty sure they were. Almost all the shrimp you can buy were, at one time or another, frozen. So, whether or not your shrimp are currently frozen, take my word for it, it's a good bet that they were.

Next plop the shrimp in boiling water for a few minutes. Remove, let cool, peel, and, pinching your nostrils closed, place the shrimp in your mouth, chew, and swallow.

It doesn't taste like much, does it? If you didn't know it was a shrimp beforehand, would anything have led you to guess correctly?

Repeat the experiment. This time don't hold your nose.

It tastes about the same? Or, to put it another way, both have zero FPC.

The shrimp that we buy in the market are almost all farm-raised, bred not for flavor but, rather, for texture and shape. They are meant to have flavor added in the form of breadings and sauces, which are high in calories, sugar, salt, white flour, and fat.

Then there are the shrimp we discovered last year at Captain Frank's, just beside Route 95 in Boynton Beach, Florida, where we shop for fish whenever we visit with my folks at the ancestral condo in West Palm Beach. Captain Frank's is a classic old seafood store, right down to the nautical bric-a-brac décor. In season, we always celebrate our last night in Florida with stone crabs. Hard-shelled, firm-fleshed, with meat that is sweeter and more buttery-tasting than the blue crabs of Maryland or even the best hard-shell lobsters from Nova Scotia. Served cold with a creamy mustard sauce, and washed down with a Sancerre or an Albariño, they are spectacular. They are also expensive, but that's when I tell myself that a restaurant meal with lesser ingredients would cost more.

"Would you like them cracked?" the woman behind the counter asked.

Unless you've got demolition equipment in your kitchen, precracked is the way to go.

I said yes, and to kill time while she went to work on our crabs, I looked over the seafood case. The local catch was gorgeous. Swordfish from Key West, glistening with a pale-pink blush like happy-hour clouds riding above a cocktail deck in the Lower Keys. Also on display were flounder, with the grayish tinge that proclaims it was recently hauled from the ocean; thick too, not the tepid white-fleshed fillets that are foisted off as freshly caught flounder in most seafood markets. Most wonderful of all, similarly gray-tinged shrimp identified by a handwritten little placard that bore the legend "Cape Canaveral Shrimp."

Fresh wild shrimp . . . never frozen . . . and from local waters. To me this was almost as miraculous as an apparition of Saint Andrew, the patron saint of fishermen. To show you how rare this has become, once, in the Florida Keys, while fishing for tarpon, I offered to make a shrimp dish for dinner. It seemed like a no-brainer—there are plenty of shrimp caught and sold in the Keys. But after an hour of driving from fish stand to grocery store to supermarket, I was ready to throw in the towel. All the shrimp in all the stores had been frozen, which does wonders for retarding spoilage but wreaks havoc on texture and upsets the finely tuned and subtle balance of flavors found in fresh-from-the-ocean shrimp. In desperation, I stopped by the local bait stand and picked up a few pounds of live Keys shrimp. They were tiny, and hell to clean . . . but so delicious.

The Cape Canaveral shrimp in Captain Frank's display case were like those Keys crustaceans, only five times as big. I bought two pounds of them, and, for good measure, two half-pound fillets of flounder.

Back at my parents' house, I put a pair of skillets on the stove: one for shrimp, one for flounder. I oiled them both (extra-virgin for such pristine seafood). First the shrimp went in, with a rat-a-tat sizzle. Two minutes later, I flipped them and threw in two minced cloves of garlic. Then I added the flounder—which had been lightly seasoned with a little kosher salt—to the other oiled skillet. In a few minutes, the shrimp were nicely red, with little browned bits, and the flounder—pleasingly firm—was likewise lightly browned.

"That's it?" my dad asked, doubtfully. But he needn't have fretted. The shrimp came out soft and sweet, the flounder delicately savory. The nutty pan-roasted garlic balanced the subtle but pleasing iodine note of fresh seafood.

For my own edification, I boiled a shrimp and performed the test of holding my nose and tasting. It was unmistakably shrimp. Then, without holding my nose, I tasted again. . . . POW! Shrimp to the tenth power, and then some.

There is simply no substitute for fresh, wild seafood. Not only is it delicious, but study after study points to its role in a balanced and healthful diet. There is little to none of the unhealthy fat that can characterize land animals raised for food under industrial conditions. We eat more and more fresh fish in restaurants, but we don't cook very much of it at home. Why?

I did my own little survey about fish cooking at a terrific meal at The Boathouse Restaurant in Charleston, South Carolina. It featured all locally caught and sustainable fish: shrimp, snapper, amberjack, wreckfish.

I went from table to table with the chef, asking folks about their meals. All forty diners oohed and aahed over the seafood. But when I asked if they made fish at home—apart from breading and deep-frying—none of them did.

"It's too easy to ruin" was the universal response, or words to that effect. The customers liked ordering it in restaurants, but felt insecure about preparing it at home. They are wrong. Fish is easy to cook.

There is also a cultural obstacle to fish consumption: the teachings of the Church. Even though meatless Fridays are no longer Catholic dogma, for two thousand years Western culture was steeped in the belief that fish was a penance and meat was a carnal pleasure. Penance may get you into heaven, but pleasure will get you through your next meal. Meat is what the Western diet points us toward even when the nearby waters are full of fish.

No doubt part of the explanation is that, as with much fresh food, after a short time fish loses texture and flavor. Worse, it smells "fishy"—i.e., the oils in salmon, cod, and tuna, for example, oxidize, even turning rancid on exposure to air. The solution to this is to buy fish that looks and smells fresh and cook it right away. How does fresh fish smell? My mentor as a fishing writer was also a great food writer, the late A. J. McClane. He advised me, "When you handle it and then sniff your hands, you should smell fresh cucumbers."

Another problem with fish is that half the seafood we consume is farmed, and although there have been strides in the quality of farm-raised seafood, much farmed fish—like feed-lot livestock—is raised on a regimen designed to put on weight quickly, with little regard for flavor. And then there are the antibiotics that are as necessary when raising fish in close quarters as they are for pigs raised in confinement.

As with livestock, there are farms that produce delicious and wholesome fish and ones that don't. Talk with the seafood manager at your supermarket, or look online at Web sites to see what they have to say about wild and farmed food. The Blue Ocean Institute (blueocean.org), CleanFish (cleanfish.com), and the Monterey Bay Aquarium (montereybayaquarium.org/cr/seafoodwatch.aspx) are reliable. Retailers such as Whole Foods have instituted a rigorous program for certifying farmed fish. Actually, so has Walmart. After one purchase, your sense of taste will tell you how well the promise is delivered on the plate. Some of these retailers sell sustainably harvested wild fish, too, which is a good thing, but it may be frozen. Freezing turns the delicate protein to mush, and there is no way to restore its texture.

Bottom line, I encourage you to eat more fish and to prepare it at home, but it is also vital that you keep the environmental and conservation issues surrounding wild seafood in mind. They are too profound to ignore.

In broad strokes, the problem is clear-cut: more people are using more technology to catch more fish out of oceans that are more environmentally stressed. The result has been declining fish stocks, destruction of habitat, and, according to a widely quoted study in the journal *Science,* oceans that will be fished out by the year 2048 unless something is done to reverse these alarming trends.

In terms of pure killing power, today's ocean hunters are light-years ahead of the buckskin-clad hunters who cleared the Great Plains of eighty million bison in the closing decades of the nineteenth century. Present-day wild-capture fishermen are more lethally equipped than Buffalo Bill with his repeating rifle, and much more efficient: armed with GPS, spotter planes, sonar, long lines, and nets that can scour miles of ocean.

The lordly bluefin tuna, pound for pound the most valuable (read: expensive) food animal on the planet, is on the path to extinction. Sushi has done this fish no favors. Species that were once ignored, such as orange roughy and Patagonian toothfish—also known as Chilean sea bass—have been nearly exterminated. Likewise, with the advent of seagoing fish-processing factories, the population of Atlantic cod, which was the finny foundation of empires, completely collapsed. After two decades of stringent conservation, we are beginning to see signs of sustainable cod recovery, although the jury is still out on whether it will ever fully come back.

The good news is that nature is often resilient. All creatures are apt to mate and multiply, so in the last twenty years we have seen the robust resurgence of striped bass on the East Coast and redfish in the Gulf of Mexico.

We have been given an opportunity that humanity last had ten thousand years ago, with the domestication of livestock. As more and more of the earth was devoted to rearing a few animal species, the diversity of living things suffered. We eliminated species and destroyed habitats. Only the creatures of the oceans persisted in something like their original diversity. We have the chance for a do-over in the seas that we are unlikely to see again on the land.

So, yes, eat fish, but vary it. Give the big guys a break, and don't keep going back to the same old tuna, salmon, cod, and striped bass that dominate most menus. If you live near a coast, you can often buy or catch local fish that rarely make it to restaurant kitchens, but because they are local and fresh, they are often equal, if not superior, in taste to salmon or cod. In my region, the much-maligned bluefish (which, when eaten fresh, has a bright and clear flavor), blackfish, and weakfish (elsewhere known as sea trout or speckled trout) are available in fish markets. I eat them seasonally, just as I do fruits and vegetables. If you don't know what is in season, look for the words "local" and "wild," and, failing that, ask the person behind the counter.

What tend to get overlooked, in environmental discussions and in cookbooks, are the little fish: sardines, anchovies, herring, and the like are delicious, plentiful, and loaded with heart-healthy omega-3's and satiety-inducing umami. Furthermore, because they are lower down on the food chain, their tissues accumulate less mercury and other harmful substances; when big fish eat little fish, they also consume and store many of the pollutants that the little fish ate. Fresh, canned, or cured, these little guys are available everywhere all year round. Whenever I am stuck for a lunch idea, some sardines in tomato sauce suit me fine.

Shopping for delicious seafood and keeping a clear environmental conscience requires us to seek out information. There are as yet not enough common standards to simplify the search, but before we buy fish at the market or order it in a restaurant, if enough of us ask whether the fish is farmed or wild, how and where the fish was caught or raised, then whenever we shop, the progress of the last two decades will continue. It will make a difference.

Culinary Necessities: My Larder

One of the things I love about big cities is that you can be inspired to cook a meal and then go out and shop on a daily basis. But putting the pleasures of small-scale shopping aside, sometimes I am too busy to shop, so I always keep some go-to ingredients on the shelves and in the fridge. You don't need to live in a city with charming markets and colorful food personalities behind the counter to fill your pantry. You can stock your larder with items found in any supermarket. If you don't feel like shopping on any given day, you can probably stay home and still make a satisfying meal. It's the difference between eating cold cereal over the sink and a nice lunch or dinner, on days when it's freezing, lashed with rain, pelted by hail, clobbered by a blizzard, or egg-frying hot on the sidewalks. As long as I have stocked my pantry, I know I can eat well. As is probably evident by now, I favor ingredients in the Mediterranean Diet, but if you like to cook Asian foods, the same principles hold: stay with easy-to-prepare whole foods and a lot of ingredients with high FPC.

ONIONS I use onions in more recipes than any other ingredient except salt. They soften, sweeten, caramelize, and crisp. I reach for them whenever I want some of those qualities in a recipe, which is almost always. When in doubt, use them.

ANCHOVIES Super-high in umami. Not everyone loves their strong flavor, but I find it indispensable. Great for sauces, especially with seafood and pasta. Melted in a saucepan and combined with olive oil to dress broccoli, cauliflower, Brussels sprouts, other hearty vegetables, or even as a basting sauce for roast leg of lamb. Eat with a slice of whole-grain bread, or top with sweet roasted peppers, and call it lunch.

SARDINES Packed in olive oil, mustard sauce, or tomato sauce. Eat with a whole-grain crisp bread for a satisfying lunch. Even better, add a slice of raw onion.

HERRING Pickled herring without cream sauce (but with plenty of onions) is satisfying in the same way that sardines are, and adds some pleasing tartness.

GOOD CHICKEN AND BEEF STOCKS Great for risotto, finishing pasta, glazing vegetables, enriching stews. I look at the label to confirm the absence of chemistry-lab additives.

PLAIN YOGURT I like the thick yogurt known as Greek-style. Even the zero-fat variety is thick, creamy, and high in protein, but I prefer the whole milk kind. Good with nuts and berries for lunch, or with frozen bananas and other fruits in a smoothie.

BACON There are few things that a little bacon cannot improve. The combination of salt, umami, smokiness, and funk (from aging) boosts flavor. Yes, bacon has lots of calories, but think of it as a seasoning rather than a main ingredient. Thin slices of country ham, or any long-cured (hard) ham, will work just as well.

ITALIAN SAUSAGE Like bacon, sausage needn't be the main event, but a little of it, diced and crisply browned, adds flavor and satiating umami to recipes with pasta, chickpeas, lentils, or couscous. We always keep some in the freezer.

BUTTER Completing my trio of surprising health foods (see Italian sausage and bacon, above), a little butter adds depth and flavor. Again, think of it as a seasoning. For example, I'll pan-roast artichokes in a few tablespoons of olive oil and then finish the process with a pat of butter. Adam Perry Lang will rub it on smoked pork shoulder for the last hour of cooking, to maintain the right balance of moisture and crispness in the precious "bark," or crust, on barbecued meat.

EGGS Free-range and organic. For breakfast, of course, but an omelet, frittata, or poached egg served with a green salad, and whole-grain toast with a drizzle of olive oil, works for lunch or dinner. When my daughter Lily was a picky eater (in her younger years), Dad's culinary exploits sometimes failed to entice her. "I'll just scramble some eggs," she would say, and that satisfied her. I get it. Eggs always satisfy.

CAPERS Salty and tart. Use them in any dressing or sauce that calls for lemon or vinegar and salt. I love to crisp them with sautéed shallots and use as a topping for fish or cold meat.

ROASTED SWEET RED PEPPERS When I was a little boy, our neighbor Sidney Shamis (who was a professor of engineering at NYU) used to shop at an old family-run Italian grocery store in Orange, New Jersey. He always returned with some of these peppers in his bag. I loved looking at all the packages with Italian words on them. Sidney's grocery bag was as close as I would get to Europe until I was in college. I put peppers on sandwiches with leftover meat, chicken, or fish, to add color and dress up a plate while contributing flavor. They're also nice with a slice of milder cheese.

A HUNK OF PARMESAN CHEESE For finishing touches on salads or soups. Use with eggs, beans, lentils, pasta. Save the rinds to enrich sauces and soups. Super-high FPC, super-high umami. Always grate your own. The pregrated stuff is like packaged peeled fruit or vegetables: it loses flavor quickly.

OLIVE OIL Do you need good olive oil for cooking? Yes, but not necessarily the most expensive. To dress salads, finish soups, or drizzle on meat or fish, use the best extra-virgin you can afford. Good olive oil has a floral aroma. I am not a big fan of spicy olive oils in general, but the balance between fruitiness and pepperiness in Spanish Arbequina adds up to a very nice all-purpose olive oil. By all means, shop for other types of olive oil. As with wine, so much good product has come on the market in recent years, you can choose from many fine oils.

CRUSHED RED-PEPPER FLAKES Heat wakes up tired ingredients and makes good ones even more flavorful. I like bottled hot sauces, but they are strongly flavored. Red-pepper flakes add heat but don't mess with taste.

FLAKY SEA SALT It tastes the same as regular table salt, which is no surprise; they are the same chemical substance. What's different is that the process of extracting this salt from the evaporation of seawater produces flakes, so that, when you use it to finish any recipe, the salt doesn't dissolve. You get concentrated bits of saltiness, and the fun of an extra element of crunch.

BEANS, LENTILS, CHICKPEAS, WHOLE-GRAIN COUSCOUS, FARRO
All of these dry ingredients can be the basis of a meal. They have a fairly long shelf life, so whenever you are stuck for an idea they are a dependable place to begin. Soak beans and chickpeas overnight, or quick-soak by boiling for 2 minutes, removing from heat, and leaving in hot water, covered, for an hour. Cook with stocks, tomatoes, Parmesan rind (or any combination of these). Toss with leftover vegetables, meat, fish, or poultry. I have at least two dinners based on these ingredients each week (which also leaves me two meals' worth of leftovers). I prefer to prepare dried ingredients from scratch,

with the possible exception of chickpeas; the canned or jarred ones from Spain are often better than my home attempts.

HARD DURUM-SEMOLINA PASTA It is smooth and slithery, and sauces cling to it in a way that they rarely if ever do to whole-grain pasta. Cook al dente, serve in four-ounce portions, and add wilted greens, browned sausage bits, chickpeas, leftover meat or fish. Really load it up with these other ingredients, especially vegetables—at least equal in volume to the pasta.

FARRO PASTA Of all the whole-grain pastas, farro comes closest in texture and sauce-clingability to hard durum-semolina. Serve with stronger-tasting sauces, wilted greens, bacon.

GOOD-TASTING WHOLE-GRAIN BREAD Beware of health breads that list "wheat flour" or "unbleached wheat flour" as the first ingredient. It needs to have "whole grain" or "whole wheat" leading the list. It took me a while to find a whole-wheat bread that I love. It's made by a baker who sells at the little Sunday farmers' market in my neighborhood, so that may not do you much good. My only advice is, keep looking and trying. You'll find one.

WHOLE-GRAIN CRACKERS, THICK CRUNCHY WASA BREAD, OR THINNER, EQUALLY CRUNCHY AK-MAK Eat with cheese, anchovies, roasted peppers, all types of pickles, cold cuts. Wasa are my favorites, but there are many whole-grain choices.

CAPONATA Canned or in jars, an eggplant-based salad, usually made with olives, onions, tomatoes. Huge flavor. A good vegetable side dish with cheese and bread or crackers.

GREENS Wilted spinach, kale, chard, and escarole are easy to prepare and high in nutrients. Always have some on hand, and always throw some in with soups, risottos, pastas.

APPLES In the fall, buy local apples. For most of the winter, there's no choice other than apples from distant climes. Fujis, Honey Crisps, and Galas tend to keep their crispness longest. The sweetness, bulk, and crunch of apples satisfy quickly.

BLUEBERRIES Beginning in May and all through the summer, blueberries are in season somewhere. Although I am not a nutrient chaser—in other words, I don't eat things solely because they have antioxidants, or a certain vitamin—I have read so many good things about blueberries, and they are a whole food, so I figure there's no downside. The upside is their super taste. Organic cost more, but I prefer them if possible. Rinse thoroughly, especially with nonorganic berries: they are commonly treated with pesticides. I also love strawberries, raspberries, and blackberries.

DRIED CRANBERRIES Good balance of bitter, fruity, and sweet. When there are no fresh berries to be had, I eat them at breakfast with almonds and whole-grain cereal, or for lunch with thick yogurt and almonds.

DRIED PRUNES, FIGS, CHERRIES Loads of flavor, great with a handful of almonds for a satisfying snack. I am particularly fond of prunes mixed in with steel-cut Irish oatmeal and farm-fresh yogurt and a drizzle of real maple syrup.

ROASTED ALMONDS Pleasing crunch, healthful fats, nice flavor, satiating protein. When I am hungry, I eat about a dozen.

They are lovely with dried cranberries and a piece of dark chocolate. This combination satisfies just about every flavor craving, and they calm my appetite. Raw almonds are fine, but I find that the roasted ones have more FPC.

ROASTED PEANUTS, CASHEWS, PECANS For all the reasons I like almonds, I like these nuts as well. I take 'em straight—no cranberries, no chocolate. I am agnostic on the salt/no-salt issue. The problem with nuts is that they pack a lot of calories, so pace yourself, which is difficult with salted nuts.

DARK CHOCOLATE OR DARK CHOCOLATE WITH CACAO NIBS Chocolate is a whole food. Just a little satisfies my sweet tooth. I was pleased to learn that Dr. Arthur Agatston, father of the South Beach Diet, is, like me, a regular chocolate consumer. I am a fan of Scharffen Berger, but there are many other fine brands. Your choice.

Your larder may vary from mine. Maybe you prefer walnuts to almonds, or raspberries to blueberries. Moreover, if I cooked only with the ingredients in this chapter, I'd get very bored and soon fall off the healthy-eating wagon. But a larder is not a diet; rather, it represents building blocks that can form the basis for many meals, changing with the seasons. You will still want fresh produce and probably some animal protein (winged, hoofed, finned, or shelled). What a larder does is guarantee that you always have some trusted ingredients on hand, ones that will help satisfy you so you won't always start from square one in the "What should I eat?" department. CI in the larder, plus a little bit of shopping, will set you up fine. And from time to time, forget the shopping and get inventive with what's on hand.

Labels

No matter how strong your resolve to eat whole, local, sustainable food, there is no getting around the reality that at every supermarket—or corner grocery, for that matter—a substantial amount of products come in a package. More often than not, the contents are not visible. The only way to apply CI when shopping for packaged goods is to read the labels.

Since all food products require a label that lists ingredients and nutritional information, you would suppose that informed consumers would never again have to eat anything without knowing what's going into their bodies. This, of course, assumes that the makers of a food want you to understand what is in their product. Don't take this on faith.

I find that one of the most confusing aspects of a food label is the nutritional information. It is always expressed according to what the manufacturer asserts is a "normal serving." But what is the definition of "normal," and who eats just a third of a cup of breakfast cereal, or just one ounce of potato chips? The percentages mean nothing to me, because I can't keep straight what 15 percent of the daily recommendation of sugar, fat, or carbs looks like. I feel like a baseball fan looking at the box score for a cricket match: all that information must mean a lot to someone, but not to me.

When I read a label, I glance at the nutritional information to get a rough idea of what kind of fat (trans fats, saturated, polyunsaturated, or monounsaturated), if any, is in the food. Then I read the ingredients to see how many times some form of sugar is listed. Often, a high level of sugar content is divvied up through such substitute words as "partially evaporated fruit sugar," "corn syrup," "pure cane sugar." My general rule here is, if sugar, in some form, appears more than once in an ingredients listing, it's too much. If there is white flour, even if it is called unbleached and organic wheat flour, I read that as sugar, because my body does.

And then there are the health claims. A package of chocolate Pop-Tarts proclaims, "One serving of whole grain and 20 percent daily value of fiber in one frosted, fudgetastic pocket of perfection." Apart from the fact that no one has ever eaten a Pop-Tart as part of a health regimen, I inherently distrust such claims. It's like when someone says, "Well, to be completely honest with you . . ." That immediately gets me wondering, "Hmm . . . what haven't you been completely honest about up to this point?" Health claims on labels are a cause for suspicion.

So, if labels are so misleading, why do I say to read or at least look at them? It's not because I'm recommending, as some back-to-basics diet advisers do, that you refrain from buying anything with more than, say, five ingredients. I am not opposed to multiple ingredients per se. Eggplant caponata, one of my favorite flavorful light lunch foods, has the following ingredients: eggplant, olive oil, onion, garlic, celery, tomatoes, capers, pine nuts, sugar, red wine vinegar, dried chili flakes, salt, olives. That's a lot, but they are all real, whole ingredients. If, on the other hand, the ingredient list is a blizzard of words that end in "-ite," "-ate," "-ide," "-ose," and "-ase," it might as well say that the food is nothing more than a collection of chemicals.

In an ideal world, if I weren't able to see the actual food I contemplated eating, I wouldn't buy it. For the most part, this is not possible in a supermarket. True, when I buy apples I look at each apple; likewise chicken, or onions. But there's no getting away from the fact that, in the real world, stocking your shelves and your refrigerator means you are going to have to buy stuff in boxes, cans, jars, and tubes. So by all means look at the label to get an overall idea, but don't dwell on deciphering it. If it takes more than half a minute to read, you probably don't want it.

The fundamental rule before buying and ultimately eating anything could not be simpler: Think! Think before you shop for food, even—or especially—if you need a quick snack; think while you are choosing items at the market or on a menu; think while you are cooking; and think while you are eating. Only through buying, cooking, ordering, and eating thoughtfully can you dial out the marketing noise and resist the thousand subliminal invitations to consume high-calorie, high-fat, super-sweet, chemically engineered foods. Wherever you turn they cry out, "Buy me! Eat me!"

CHAPTER IV

The Fundamentals of Flavor: The Elements of Taste

Flavor is the most ancient language. It predates music and came long before words. It carries a vital message of sustenance to every cell in our bodies. Each element of flavor is overdetermined—i.e., sensory shorthand for the effect of thousands of food components—and because of this it takes very little to completely transform a dish.

Everyone, from the gourmet chef brandishing a truffle slicer to the spoon-in-hand infant attacking a bowl of applesauce, has an inborn and highly complex sense of flavor that informs the imagination and fuels the appetite. This flavor sense helps us choose between beef and pork, deep-frying versus broiling, whether to add sugar or salt. Compared with the Western musical scale with its twelve tones, the possible ways to combine the basic properties of flavor are practically infinite. There are thousands of edible plants and animals. Because the building blocks that the chef can assemble are so much greater in number than those available to the composer of songs, it is inspiring, yet at the same time daunting, to consider that you could take all the songs ever sung and still not approach the number of recipes that we humans could come up with to satisfy hunger.

We all have the capacity to understand flavor. Developing that capacity leads to a more pleasurable and healthful way of eating, much more so than denying ourselves and counting calories, or turning over control to some diet or nutrition authority and, without further thought, following a one-size-fits-all, preplanned regimen. This kind of detailed battle plan for weight loss is my problem with many diets. "On day four," one diet might prescribe, "lunch: a slice of whole-grain toast, turkey breast and avocado, green tea, blueberries with a dollop of nonfat yogurt for dessert."

My reaction: a guaranteed turnoff. Not that I have any objections to whole-grain toast. Or turkey breast, for that matter . . . Well, maybe a little problem if it's house-brand turkey, which often has the texture of sliced bologna and the chemically stoked aroma of a Burger King Whopper. Likewise, avocado is a fine fruit; yogurt is creamy, which is always nice; and having berries for dessert is okay by me. What's the problem, then? Most diets leave no room for serendipity and spontaneous inspiration. How can I possibly know what I will be in the mood for on day four, or five, or six of my new diet? Laying out a food plan as if it were the itinerary of a package tour removes one of the most stimulating pleasures of food. The question is, what do I feel like having now? Not two days or a week from now, but *now.*

Any diet that is constrained in this rigid fashion is inherently hard to follow over the long run, because it is no fun. Consuming what someone else tells you to eat may help you lose weight initially, but it is not likely to help you keep it off. How you eat and how you think about food—long-term—are your greatest allies. To be sure, there are some decisions to make about what *not* to eat, but once you take those few steps, then healthy eating is much more about seeking pleasure, and maximum taste experience. You must engage your imagination, be aware of your desires, and possess the culinary information to make decisions that will satisfy you now, because any diet is only as good as your next meal, and that next meal will only be as good as your ability to choose the right thing.

First order of business: learn to understand taste. Early in my career as a food writer, I felt that I had to do a better job of describing taste. Like many journalists, I fell back on very general terms in describing food.

"Earthy," "gutsy," "delicate," "woodsy," "briny," "smoky," "bright"—these are words that writers commonly use to communicate what a given dish tastes like. But even though these terms convey a general notion, they don't tell you much about the experience of any food in particular. Asparagus can be earthy; so can a truffle, or a carrot. Yet they are much more different in taste than they are alike. You might remark on the intense tomato flavor of one dish and the heavy presence of garlic in another. But what does tomato taste like, or garlic? Describing them in terms of themselves doesn't tell the reader much beyond what one can easily surmise from a list of ingredients. Much more useful, or at least informative, is a description of the flavor of a tomato that tells you it is acidic (tangy), balanced with sweetness, that it has umami, or that its juicy flesh is as smooth in texture as, say, a veal shank that has been braised to extreme unctuousness.

Restaurant critics don't as a rule delve into the inner taste logic of a dish. In fairness, they rarely have room for such speculations in a nine-hundred-word column, which was the norm when I first started reviewing; in online food writing, reviews are often shorter. Moreover, restaurant reviewing is a literary form that was basically codified by the first professional reviewer, French bon vivant Grimod de La Reynière (1758–1837), who reported on Parisian restaurants, using as his template his earlier theater reviews. In consequence, ever since that day, reviewers have written as if the restaurant experience were a performance in which ambience, clientele, and design are almost as important as food. That doesn't leave much space for a quick summing up of a half-dozen dishes in the hope that this will give readers a feel for the range of cuisine. Finally, the reviewer must save room for a clever sign-off and the meting out of stars, points, forks, or whatever system the critic uses to convey a judgment.

Discussion of the taste of food was left to generalities. In contrast, wine writers have an elaborate taste lexicon to describe just one product—fermented grape juice. As a literary form, it fairly begs to be satirized. I have nothing against connoisseurship, and wine is one of life's glories. Appreciating its nuances helps to explain and deepen the considerable pleasure locked inside a wine bottle. But where are the panegyrics to aged ham, caramelized sweet onions, crusty aged beef, dark chocolate studded with roasted almonds? Each of these foods is as complex in its own way as a bottle of Romanée-Conti.

Cookbook authors, although not limited to a word count, rarely do much better. Where the restaurant critic is constrained by space, the author of a cookbook has the opposite problem: how to fill up a book so that it has enough pages to justify the price? Even though we turn to cookbooks for recipes, a mere listing of ingredients and cooking methods would yield a work that, if no less useful, is too skimpy to earn pride of place on the coffee table.

Bulked up with photographs of dishes you'd be hard pressed to duplicate without the services of a highly paid food stylist, such books also represent the apotheosis of the headnote—150 words (often a mix of random remembrances of the chef's childhood and pro-forma paeans to seasonality) preceding the actual list of ingredients and method.

I am not arguing for less beautiful photography or less evocative writing. My books, I hope, are guilty of both. Instead, I am saying that even the most ecstatic writing and glorious images rarely tell you how something is going to taste. The three books that contributed most to my development as a home cook had zero photography. Instead, simple line drawings did the trick in Irma Rombauer's *Joy of Cooking,* Julia Child's *Mastering the Art of French Cooking,* and Sheila Lukins and Julee Rosso's *The Silver Palate Cookbook.*

Julia Child's recipes are the most bulletproof I've ever read, and Sheila Lukins opened up the world of cuisine outside of France after we had worked our way through Julia, but of the three I suppose Irma Rombauer's is the one to whom I owe the greatest debt, simply because she got me started. A large part of Rombauer's charm is her mix of the methodical and the screwball (q.v. her diagram of how to skin a squirrel, which looks like a guy in work boots attempting to undress a Barbie doll).

Like most Americans—especially those exposed to the propaganda of quick 'n' easy convenience that dominated our food culture in the postwar decades—I knew very little about how to cook apart from the mental movies I carried around from watching my mom and her mom. Although they instilled in me an appreciation for taste and texture, there was nothing I had taken from their briskets and blintzes, veal cutlets and shish kebabs, that I knew how to translate in my own kitchen. They were more like random if beautiful scenes from an unfinished movie. Rombauer was a free spirit, untrammeled by the set-in-stone strictures of contemporary cookbooks, as evidenced by my all-time favorite headnote, on page 385 of the 1975 edition of *Joy of Cooking:*

> The uninitiated are sometimes balked by the intractable appearance of a lobster at table. They may take comfort from the little cannibal who, threading his way through the jungle one day at his mother's side, saw a strange object flying overhead. "Ma, what's that?" he quavered. "Don't worry, sonny," said Ma. "It's an airplane. Airplanes are pretty much like lobsters. There's an awful lot you have to throw away, but the insides are delicious."

Sadly, it does not appear in the most recent revision.

Even those classic books, despite their thorough step-by-step instructions, told very little about how a thing tasted. I would not know that until I actually made the recipe. A description of how ingredients interacted and to what effect would have been helpful.

I had begun to ponder the question of taste and how to explain it when I met Gray Kunz at a chefs' outing in the Catskills. At the time he enjoyed a reputation as one of the top three or four chefs in the world. He is a kitchen polymath, at home in four of the world's richest culinary cultures. Of European background, Kunz was raised in Singapore with its rich heritage of Indian and South Asian food. He trained in Switzerland, apprenticed under Frédy Girardet (at that time Michelin's top-rated chef), and worked six years as a chef in Hong Kong. This is all by way of saying that before the term "fusion cuisine" came into common use, Kunz—by virtue of his upbringing—had an intimate acquaintance with the cuisines of India, China, Southeast Asia, and Europe.

New York restaurant-goers in the 1980s and '90s were eager for new flavors and fine-dining elegance. Gray found himself in the right place at the right time. It didn't hurt that the St. Regis Hotel threw a fortune at its in-house restaurant, Lespinasse, in the hope that by domiciling a great chef they would attract well-heeled international travelers as well as New York's masters of the financial universe.

A few weeks after I first met Gray, Bryan Miller, who had recently relinquished his position as restaurant critic for the *New York Times,* joined Melinda and me for one of Kunz's tasting menus at Lespinasse.

Our meal was varied, surprising, novel, audacious. It included a salad of peekytoe crabs and melon, sautéed foie gras with lentils and quince, braised salmon in a Syrah-wine reduction, roast rack of lamb in a carrot emulsion, his signature braised short ribs, strawberry-and-champagne soup with grapefruit sherbet, chocolate-banana soufflé.

"That was the best meal I have had in five years," the hard-to-impress Miller declared.

"I'll see you and raise you, Bryan," I said. "That was the best meal I ever had."

I often say this whenever I have a truly great meal. Never mind that it is logically impossible—they can't *all* be the best meal ever. But in the immediate post-dining flush of pleasure that follows such an experience, you honestly believe that it is true. A great chef, home or professional, can make you feel that way.

I left the restaurant that night with a book idea taking shape. Every one of Gray's dishes impressed me with how it combined flavors and textures. Each mouthful told its own short story with a beginning, a middle, and an end.

I let the memory of that meal marinate in my mind until, a few weeks later, I approached Gray with an idea for a cookbook based on different tastes. Rather than the classic cookbook organization of appetizer, soup, fish, poultry, meat, vegetable, dessert, I suggested that we build our book around tastes. Please note, in conversation I often use the words "taste" and "flavor" interchangeably. For purposes of more acute analysis, scientists speak of "tastes" as those elements for which we have taste receptors on our palates, whereas "flavor" takes in the whole world of aroma, heat, texture: the total experience of the sensual properties of any food.

But what are the characteristics of the fundamental tastes? For such a basic aspect of life necessary to our survival, there is very little written. Food scientists have published numerous studies on such arcana as "Enantiomeric Specificity of Alanine Taste Receptor Sites in Catfish" (*Brain Research,* 1987) or "Quantitative Anatomical Study of Taste Buds in Fungiform Papillae of Young and Old Fischer Rats" (*Journal of Gerontology,* 1986), but these academic works, however well founded, don't really tell me, for example, how salt affects the crunchy crust of a pan-roasted steak.

Over the next few months, Gray and I tasted and analyzed hundreds of ingredients: apples and anchovies, pomegranates and prosciutto, morels and mozzarella, turnips and tarragon, Cherry Garcia and cheddar cheese, Vietnamese fish rolls and Vermont venison, duck breast, beef cheeks, frogs' legs, chicken wings, veal feet, and pigs' knuckles. We came up with a system for understanding what the basic tastes are and how they interact. We tasted ingredients and tested recipes with a cross section of people—third-graders, grandparents, professional cooks, people who couldn't even fry an egg, fashion models, portly businessmen, any available neighbor, the guy who came to fix the air conditioner, the mailman.

The surprising thing was how often this disparate sample of humanity agreed. Or maybe it's not so surprising. As I said at the outset of this chapter, our sense of taste is a highly evolved and complex system of shorthand that attracts us to the foods that can best sustain us. For want of a system that put this into words, Gray and I devised our own language of taste. It continues to help me to be a better cook and a smarter eater.

The Elements of Taste

It has been nearly fifteen years since Gray and I began work on our book. Though I've tried to refine and simplify our framework over time, in its basics it still serves to help me to understand how a dish works and to make decisions on what to cook, how to shop, what to choose in a restaurant. So, even though butter, cream, sugar, chunks of sausage, melted cheese, and a crispy crust fried in calorie-rich oil could possibly make a lump of granite taste good, there are other ways to pump up the flavor and satisfaction you get from food. Once you take the time to understand what you are eating (and cooking), you will enjoy it more and have a better-quality diet, one that can satisfy without defaulting to instantly fattening ingredients.

When chefs talk about balancing a sauce (and they all do), they mean they are going to adjust sweetness (usually sugar or honey), saltiness, tartness (lemon juice, wine, vinegar), and heat (black pepper, chili pepper, ginger, horseradish). These are the basics. Any one of them will complement the effect of all the other flavor components in a dish. Remove them and the primest prime rib is dull and flaccid, ice cream becomes congealed cold milk, and a hearty chili is just boiled beans. These basic tastes can always be combined to create a fuller-flavored dish: salt in a chocolate-chip cookie, sugar and crushed red-pepper flakes in marinara sauce. They also share another characteristic: once added, they cannot be taken away. It is true that you can balance one taste with another, but it is equally true that too much salt is too much salt, and balancing it with sugar will only end up with a dish that is both too salty and too sweet.

SALT

Salt is the king of tastes. As Norwegian author Frans Bengtsson wrote in his Viking epic *The Long Ships,* "There is nothing like salt. . . . A man should eat all the salt he can. It gives health and strength and long life. It drives bad things from the body and makes the blood good and fresh. Everybody likes salt."

Although modern humans can usually count on a reliable supply of salt, we still crave it the way our more deprived ancestors did in 25,000 B.C. Charles Leslie, under whom I studied anthropology in graduate school, once estimated that we probably consume twelve thousand times more salt than our Paleolithic forebears.

I always use kosher (coarse) salt for seasoning soups and stews. To salt something just before serving, I keep a supply of flaky sea salt (such as Maldon salt or *fleur de sel*). Not only does it liven up flavor, but because it doesn't dissolve instantly it provides little islands of saltiness, for an interesting contrast to the surface of the food that lies in between those islands. Think of flaky salt as creating "geography," because it localizes salty flavor wherever it lands, rather than adding a uniform coating of saltiness. It also adds crunchiness, which is almost always a good thing. As for very fine salt, I normally don't use it. It's okay for soups and stews, I guess, but it just feels too uniform and refined to me.

SWEET

All human beings are born with a sweet tooth—with good reason. Sugar equals energy. In fact, even before we have teeth, our first food, breast milk, is sweet. We find sugar in many highly nutritious foods, particularly fruits. In season, sugar-rich foods are abundant and were therefore easy for our forebears to gather. It takes a lot of sugar for sweetness to register on our taste receptors, because only a high concentration of sugar indicates food with high energy. That is why ripe fruits have such full flavor and fruits that are picked before they are ripe have little or no taste. Not only do they lack sweetness, but, without sugar to push them forward, their other flavors won't come into play nearly as forcefully. Think of the strong hint of vanilla and gardenia in a ripe peach, but never in one that is picked too soon. Sugar brings out grace notes that make for subtle, complex, and full flavor.

Sweetness rounds out the sharp edges of aromatic spices such as cloves or the tartness of lemon. It also helps other flavors to play nicely with one another; or, to borrow a musical term, sugar, when used in proportion, promotes harmony.

One of my favorite foods, chocolate, exemplifies how sugar can make something pleasantly sweet but not sugary to the point of vibrating your fillings. If you look at the label of many commercial chocolate bars—even premium ones that ballyhoo fair trade and saving the rain forests—sugar is often the first or second ingredient listed. Given the bitter, tannic taste of cacao nibs (found inside the seeds), which are the raw material for chocolate, some sugar is required to make it palatable.

But according to champagne-producer-turned-chocolate-maker John Scharffenberger, his Holy Grail is a recipe for chocolate that calls for hardly any sugar. He has devoted years to his quest. Every so often his FedEx deliveries contain a sampling of magical beans from some small farmers thousands of miles away. This was the case with the pale cacao beans he received from the small village of Tzalamtun, in the highlands of Guatemala. To use John's winemaker vocabulary, the smooth flavor of this cacao had "very soft tannins."

On assignment for *Condé Nast Traveler,* I accompanied John on a trip to meet the cacao growers of Tzalamtun. Up to that point, all of Scharffenberger's communications with the village had been via Internet, apparently going through an attorney in the nearby city of Cobán.

To reach the isolated village, we made our way along a highway that ran next to a rushing river, swollen with the floods of February. We crossed it on a ferry attached to a cable and propelled by a hand-cranked winch. Six more miles of bone-rattling four-wheel-driving along a muddy track brought us to our destination. We met in the village longhouse. John communicated through an interpreter who spoke English and Spanish, and then relayed through another interpreter who spoke Spanish and one of the twenty-three Mayan languages, related to but not the exact Kekchi Mayan spoken in that village. Waiting for a simple question to make its way through this chain of tongues was reminiscent of the scene in *Lost in Translation* in which a wacky Japanese TV director speaks at great length to Bill Murray only to have his animated discourse distilled down to a yelp or grunt.

Still, the message got through. Scharffenberger offered to pay the villagers the world-market rate—which was nearly 700 percent more than they were accustomed to receiving from the first of a series of middlemen. His reasoning was that it would cost him no more than he was already paying, and it would dissuade the Indians from cutting down the rain forest to raise corn when they could realize much more income from growing cacao, which requires the shade of the rain forest to flourish.

"Where's Pablo?" John said, and then, by way of further identification, "You know, the lawyer I have been e-mailing."

"Lawyer? You mean my son?" the *cacique* (headman) said. "He's sixteen years old and lives in Cobán. He's the only one of us who knows how to work a computer."

We all had a good laugh and then adjourned to the cookhouse, where an old woman proceeded to grind cacao on a *metate* (stone grinder), occasionally dousing the pulverized nibs with water, until she produced a paste that looked like cocoa. She heated the liquid over a wood fire and ladled it into cups, leaving us to do our own sweetening.

"If I add just a little bit of sugar, it is smooth and balanced," John said. "That tells me that to make chocolate from these beans you wouldn't need very much sugar at all. Maybe you could make delicious chocolate that is almost ninety percent pure cacao!"

This is a sensible approach to using sugar, almost as a seasoning rather than a main ingredient. In a similar vein, Gray Kunz used to refer to "chefs' desserts." By that he meant you can create a dessert by starting with a savory flavor, then adding sugar to the point that it is noticed. This is the opposite of starting, as dessert chefs often do, with sugar and adding other flavors until they rise above the pervasive sweetness.

SPICY HEAT

Spicy heat is not a taste per se. There are no taste buds for it. Instead, it activates pain receptors on the tongue, the same ones that detect warmth. But, like the true basic tastes, it has an immediate, noticeable effect, which happens in the mouth, elevating all the other tastes in a recipe. Leave it out and the dish may be nothing special.

Take my grandma Lena's "fillet of flunder." I was a teenager before it dawned on me that "flunder" was just her Eastern European way of saying "flounder." Lena was a great cook. Using a battered old steel pan on a gas stove, she served a simple yet sublime fried egg in brown butter, with a buttered hard roll to mop up the runny yolk. Her recipe for pot roast, though unorthodox, was equally memorable: "Put the pot roast and some onions in a pot and brown them until you can smell them burning in the store downstairs. Run up the stairs and add half a cup of water. Turn down the heat and cover the pot." Result: a perfect pot roast, and, it should be noted, a technique for umami extraction identical to, though neither so laborious nor so refined as, Escoffier's classic *glace de viande* (concentrated meat stock).

Her one consistent miss was her "flunder." Made with onions, carrots, and tomatoes, it lacked personality. I ranked it just above liver and onions, a notorious kid nonfavorite. However, as I discovered on an assignment in Cajun country, something as simple as changing one ingredient can make all the difference in a taste experience. Consider the fish stew that Cajuns call "gaspergou courtbouillon" (coo-boo-YAHN).

Gaspergou, the local name of a freshwater relative of the redfish, is a silly-sounding Dr. Seuss kind of word, just right for this phlegmatic creature, which I found to be dim-witted even by fish standards. Whereas other fish put up a ferocious fight when hooked, and they often succeed in breaking free, Monsieur

Gaspergou displays the fish version of Stockholm syndrome: he is very cooperative.

There is probably no better place for an introduction to this traditional dish than in the wild heart of Cajun country, the Atchafalaya Basin, where a branch of the Mississippi overflows its banks to flood five thousand square miles of fertile lowlands. It's everything you'd ever hope to see in a swamp: bald cypress trees vaulting over watery avenues, and Spanish moss hanging from tree limbs like ticker tape confetti streamers. In the black waters, you'll see alligators, snakes, otters, beaver, and minklike nutria.

Twenty generations of French-speaking Louisianans have come here to hunt deer, duck, and turkey and to catch bass, catfish, and gaspergou. Among the daily visitors at the time of my visit were commercial fisherman Connie Serrette and his business partner Alan Zeringue, a retired Mississippi riverboat pilot who had pushed barges full of gasoline, salt, and sulfur from New Orleans all the way to St. Paul. Serrette and Zeringue, like every Cajun—man, woman, and perhaps child—can cook. Nearly all Cajuns have fishing and hunting camps that they go to whenever they can. Some of these camps are nicer than a well-kept house, and some are just shacks in small clearings. The interior of Serrette's rambling green-sided camp was typical: trophy deer antlers, turkey feathers, a rack of beat-up shotguns, and black-and-white photos of long-departed swampers with wide grins as they posed with fish, deer, and waterfowl they had taken. Also, the *de rigueur* Old Black Pot—elsewhere known as a cast-iron Dutch oven.

For all its depth of flavor, this court bouillon is a deceptively simple recipe. First step, season the fish with salt and pepper—not white pepper, not black pepper, but fiery cayenne, as much as you think you can stand, and then some more. Next sweat some onions, bell peppers, and celery. Then pour in two cups of crushed tomatoes, let the liquid cook down, and, finally, add the fish, to cook about ten minutes. The finished dish was light yet with bright powerhouse flavor. When I handed the recipe in along with my story, the report back from the *Food & Wine* test kitchen was fulsome in its praise. They absolutely loved it.

Two dishes—Grandma's flunder and the Cajuns' gaspergou—almost the same, but while the flunder was forgettable, the gaspergou was delicious. The difference? Cayenne.

Just one sensation—spicy heat—elevated this way of making fish from an "I'm Not Hungry" ranking to "Please May I Have Some More?" Nothing complicated or fancy, yet one recipe was superb and the other sub par, which is why I believe that time spent on learning about taste can increase your enjoyment of food and help you to make better choices when shopping, cooking, or ordering in a restaurant.

Even though it boosts flavor, the fiery effect of chili peppers, cayenne, horseradish, wasabi, and ginger is not to everyone's liking. I have found that the world is divided into two kinds of people. There are those who like spicy food and those who say, "I like it spicy but not *too* spicy." Translation: "I despise spicy food!" When asked if they want to go to a Mexican or Thai restaurant, such folks will feign a lack of concern when offhandedly inquiring, "Is the food very spicy?" adding, "Not that I care a lot, just curious." They do care a lot. Put it this way: people who are not bothered by spicy food never ask this question. The fact of the matter is, nobody is born liking spicy food. We must learn to like it.

I was not brought up on spicy food. I developed a taste for it in Mexico City, when I was a gofer with the production company that made the Rocky and Bullwinkle cartoons. It was the summer after my freshman year in college. I lived in a small apartment at Tejocotes 10 in the Colonia del Valle neighborhood. Across the street was a Moskvitch car dealership where these Soviet-era, boxy, underpowered, and mechanically unreliable autos were sold. For three months the same forlorn little car, with its drab beige paint job, gathered dust in the showroom. I don't think they ever actually made a sale. The only activity I observed occurred each afternoon, when a pig who resided in the adjoining yard wallowed in a wet spot under the car dealer's downspout.

The occupant of the other apartment on my floor was Arturo Imaz Garza, a former millionaire who had retired to a ranch in Baja only to have things go bad when his entire herd died off from hoof-and-mouth disease. In spite of this, Arturo retained a sunny disposition, no doubt in part because he had a very sweet girlfriend named Doris who stood by him (after the wife and his other girlfriends deserted his sinking financial ship). It was the first time in my life that I had to cook for myself on a regular basis. I learned a lot from Arturo and Doris: how to prepare the week's frijoles (with chili peppers), how to make guacamole with fresh mountain herbs (and chili peppers), how to make tomatillo salsa (with chili peppers again), huevos à la mexicana (which are scrambled eggs with chili peppers). I knew I had finally become a spicy food devotee the day we climbed the Pyramid of the Sun at the ceremonial complex of Teotihuacán, just outside Mexico City.

"Pick up some fresh string cheese at the market," Arturo instructed before we set out. "We'll take care of the rest."

Three hours later, after climbing 248 steps to the summit of the pyramid, I found out what he meant by "the rest." I unwrapped my string cheese. Doris produced a stack of fresh tortillas, and Arturo presented a bag of jalapeño peppers. That was it. No ham. No chicken. Just cheese, tortillas, and jalapeños.

I was hot and hungry. As you can imagine, the apex of a pyramid offers few food choices other than what you carry up there with you.

"Eat them, you meezerable bastard," Arturo said, using the affectionate nickname he had settled on for me.

I did as I was told and wolfed down a half-dozen peppers with cheese wrapped up in a few tortillas. *No problema.*

And so, thanks to Arturo and Doris's crash course in Spicy Eating 101, I began to learn how to deal with hot food the way everyone else does: you eat enough of it and you begin to expect it; you miss it if it's not there. But first you must suffer.

TART, TANGY, ACIDIC

Tartness, like sweetness, saltiness, and spiciness, complements the tastes in food, adding life to recipes that would be much less interesting without it: the tanginess of lemon juice, the acidity of wine or a ripe tomato, the undefined but unmistakable zing of a dash of vinegar in a ragout, balances other tastes. Without this balance, the overall taste experience can be flabby, amorphous, uncontained. Tartness frames other powerful, unruly flavors in a recipe.

I think of the other tastes as pushing the flavors in a dish forward; tartness feels as if it is *pulling* flavor. Try sucking on a piece of lemon and then biting into a freshly cooked shrimp sautéed with garlic. After an initial puckering, you feel your mouth filling with flavor, like a tire being pumped up with air. Very often tanginess is the one missing element that completes a recipe, puts a bow on it, and advertises that it is as full-flavored as it is going to get.

Sometimes the effect of tartness is completely in the background; for example, with beans or lentils, a dash of vinegar or lemon brightens up the occasional palate-deadening effect of these healthful foods. Even though tartness stays below the conscious threshold of taste, the chickpeas or white beans or lentils will wake up.

Tartness is so assertive that one tends to forget that it often serves as a mediator. When we add tartness, we can often increase saltiness or sweetness without fear that it will dominate the recipe. The net result is more overall flavor.

With many meats—which are full-flavored but have no acidity—adding a little tartness is crucial in boosting flavor, almost as important as salting. Argentina's ubiquitous chimichurri sauce (see page 233), which combines tartness, saltiness, sweetness, and an herbal aroma, is a prime example. It works with any grilled meat, fish, or poultry.

I haven't reduced it to a formula, but instinctively I sense that when you use acid as a seasoning, rather than as a dominant flavor—on a slice of roast lamb, a serving of sweetbreads, or a crispy grilled chicken—you effectively double the sensual experience of each mouthful: thus, you are satisfied with less.

In long braises and stews, the acid component of wine keeps the flavor very immediate and focused. Such recipes require acid or they become lackluster, even flabby. Because red wine has bitter tannins as well, it works hand in hand with the acid in the grapes to balance the unctuous rich meatiness of short ribs or boeuf bourguignon. In tomato sauces, white wine is transformational, adding extra tanginess to the sweet, umami, acidic taste of tomato.

Without vinegar or lemon juice, salad dressing would be an uninspiring mix of fat (oil), salt, and pepper. Tartness pulls the fresh taste of a salad together. If not for lemon juice, the sugar in apple pie, or anything based on cooked fruit, would completely dominate. Tartness, with perhaps a pinch of salt, adds just the right amount of counterpoint to a homemade pie's powerful melody of sweetness.

Taste and Harmony

The mastery of the art of mixing and balancing taste and flavor is what separates great chefs (home chefs included) from dutiful, run-of-the-mill cooks. Quite often the person with the best palate in any restaurant kitchen is the *saucier,* the person who makes the sauce that balances these tastes. The great Roger Vergé, famed for his light and delicate "cuisine of the sun," told me that he felt that Daniel Boulud truly came into his own during his time as *saucier* in Vergé's three-star Michelin restaurant, Moulin de Mougins.

In less-than-expert hands, a sauce can be an exercise in flavor overkill that disguises shortcomings in the quality of ingredients or the quality of the cook. Too many so-called gourmet restaurants drown food in thickened, butter-rich, fruity, wine-soaked sauces that demolish any intrinsic flavors of the main ingredient. To do this to a great cut of meat, or slowly caramelized vegetables, is like wallpapering over the *Mona Lisa* in an attempt to improve it.

A balanced sauce will enhance, focus, and strengthen the main flavors in a recipe, not mask them. It is never enough merely to make a sauce that tastes good when you sample a spoonful of it by itself. You have to think ahead to the effect of the sauce in combination with the food being sauced. It follows from this that a good sauce will inevitably taste overseasoned on its own—it needs to be, in order to play its part when added to the larger mélange of flavors in a recipe. It must shout in order to be noticed.

A good chef understands this and can execute. I am a reasonably good home chef. Still, my palate is much less educated than that of a restaurant chef. For all I know, we may have the same natural ability, but as in learning to play an instrument or swing a golf club, practice and repetition are indispensable to mastering the art of cuisine.

I was given firsthand proof of this a few years ago, when *Food & Wine* approached me with a high-concept cooking caper: take one food-loving family (mine), give them a book by the world's reigning French chef (Alain Ducasse), and ask them to make lunch from his recipes. Then, just to make things interesting, invite the chef over to taste the results.

I wasn't afraid of cooking for a culinary big shot: I have found over the years that chefs are pretty easy to please when they are off duty. After all, the reason they are in the business in the first place is that they like food. A good steak or a well-fried chicken can charm the stars off the most demanding chef. In this regard, my mom is fond of telling the story of how she was in a tizzy over having to cook something for Jacques Pépin (who was a close friend of our family friend Gloria Zimmerman, a wonderful writer and cook). "Make me a hamburger," he said, "and I will like it. I love hamburgers."

When I received the request for the "Do It Yourself Ducasse" story, we were spending August in a rental cabin in the Adirondacks. A few days after I told *Food & Wine* I'd look into their idea, Ducasse's latest cookbook arrived. It called for lots of truffles and foie gras. As a cookbook that an average person might cook from, I thought it was inaccessible. There's nothing wrong with these jewels of Gascon cuisine. I love fresh truffles—foie gras too—but in Lake Placid you are not likely to find either of them in the supermarket. For that matter, they are not in the market in my neighborhood in New York City either.

"I think I'll pass," I began to write my editor, but then recalled seeing one of Ducasse's books, *Flavors of France,* which had a few intriguing and—as I remembered them—not impossible recipes. I asked that a copy be sent to me. It arrived shortly, and I began to page through it. My goal was to find recipes that would make an interesting meal with ingredients that I could find in the Grand Union in Lake Placid.

With a few swaps (for example, using the syrup from canned cherries combined with vinegar in place of the cherry vinegar called for by Ducasse), the ingredients list did not pose an insurmountable challenge for an American supermarket. My younger daughter, Lily, who was ten at the time, picked out a pear bread that she worked through with ease. She has always been a good baker. Her big sister, Lucy, breezed through jasmine-tea crème brûlée (custard infused with tea and a burnt-sugar crust), and Melinda made a tomato tartlet. It was August, and the tomatoes were perfect: juicy, almost smoky-tasting, and tangy. We did a dry run in the teeny kitchen in our cabin. To the peaceful serenade of a loon on the nearby West Branch of the Ausable, we ate it all, and felt confident we could reproduce it back home in the city.

I gave *Food & Wine* the thumbs-up. They rented a loft in Manhattan, perhaps intended to give the impression that we were a reasonably trendy New York family with a big kitchen in a light-drenched loft. Our real home is a floor-through apartment in a 170-year-old brownstone, which, though it has loads of light and charm, is not by any stretch a spacious loft with a half-acre of cooking space. If we put a center island in our kitchen, we'd have to give up a bedroom to accommodate it.

Ducasse arrived with his longtime girlfriend (they have since married), Gwénaëlle Guéguen. Although I had met the illustrious chef a number of times over the years, it was always in a restaurant setting where he comported himself with the Gallic reserve that one might take for *hauteur,* but here, in an informal lunch setting, he was at ease.

He and Gwénaëlle ate every bit of everything we put before them with no critical comments. When it came time to serve his steak recipe with its intense sauce of veal stock and a sweet-and-sour cherry reduction, I asked him, if he were making this at home, would he serve it with a Jackson Pollock swoosh of sauce across the plate and under the steak, as *Top Chef* wannabes do, or would he, like a normal civilian, spoon some over the meat?

He took that as an invitation to shed his sport coat, borrow an apron, walk over to the stove, pick up a spoon, and try the sauce. What had started as nearly a gallon of wine, vinegar, and cherry juice had been simmered and reduced to a cup and a half of intense garnet liquid.

Ducasse tasted, I watched. He closed his eyes and ticked his tongue against his palate as he absorbed and analyzed the full flavor. He added some salt and tasted again, then pepper, then more salt and more pepper, repeating this for a half-dozen assays. I had thought it quite good, but I had attempted this dish just three times, while he had made the same sauce hundreds of times, and other sauces thousands of times. He knew how a sauce should taste in the pan, and later, on the food. By fiddling with the balance of the main flavors, he had made my good sauce into a memorable one. What he did, and what I neglected to do, was to taste the sauce as if it were already being consumed with a mouthful of meat—I had merely tasted to see that it was good by itself. We don't consume sauce like soup. The trick is being able to taste ahead, so to speak, and imagine the effect of a sauce when it is eaten with the star ingredient, in this case steak. The result was sweet, savory, salty, spicy, and completely mouth-watering when eaten with a pan-roasted rib eye.

For the record, Ducasse spooned the sauce over the sliced steak, just the way they do at Applebee's.

UMAMI

Umami, which was first identified by Japanese scientists more than a century ago, often signals edible protein. All meat, fish, dairy, fruits, and vegetables have some protein, so they all have some umami. On an intellectual basis I understood this, but it wasn't until recently that I could say that I recognized it. I took my first steps after a meal at Blue Hill last summer. I found myself thinking about the intense flavor of the little swab of sauce that was served with a chicken breast. Apart from a little saltiness it had few of the taste characteristics of Ducasse's cherry sauce. Where Ducasse's creation was layered and full of different taste notes, Dan Barber's sauce struck one massive chord. Not better nor worse, just different. Very savory, with a beautiful mouth-feel. If asked to describe it more precisely, I'd fumble for words and say that it was "chickeny." Not salty, not sweet, not sour—just whatever it is that makes chicken taste like chicken. I asked Dan how he did it.

"We break the stock three times and each time we break it, we intensify."

"Dan, what the hell is breaking?" I asked.

"We reduce the stock until it breaks," he answered tautologically.

"Uh . . . well . . . uh . . ."

He sensed my bafflement. "Why don't you come by the restaurant some morning and we'll walk you through it."

Later that week, my daughter Lucy and I met Trevor Kunk, one of Dan's chefs at Blue Hill. It's a serious restaurant kitchen.

If you stand anywhere near the stovetop you can well imagine that this is what it must feel like to stoke a blast furnace.

Over the next four hours Lucy and I watched and tasted.

First Trevor made a bouillon.

It tasted like chicken soup.

Then he simmered roasted chicken bones and a caramelized onion in the strained bouillon.

It tasted like chicken soup, only more so.

He oiled a large pan and filled it with a layer of raw chicken wings and drumettes and browned them at high heat. The idea here was to get a good Maillardized crust. If you are not familiar with the Maillard reaction, it is the chemically complex process that occurs when heat, sugar, and protein interact. It is responsible for the crust that builds up on meat and some vegetables when they are subjected to heat. It is also the secret to the complex flavor of long-cured meats, such as *ibérico* ham. It is essential to getting maximum Flavor per Calorie. When Trevor was satisfied that the browning was done, he covered the bones with strained roast-chicken stock and boiled rapidly to reduce the liquid.

"We boil it to the breaking point," he said.

"Which is . . . ?"

He nudged a chicken wing away from the side of the pan. As it pulled away, the liquid had thickened so much that it reminded me of strings of mozzarella trailing off a slice of hot pizza.

We tasted again.

It was . . . hmm . . . extra chickeny.

Trevor explained, "When those strings snap, you're at the breaking point. If you let it cook further, the emulsion will separate. You need to stop just before then."

Through two more reductions, the chicken flavor grew ever

more profound. The final reduction reproduced the magical sauce that I had asked Dan about. No added acid or sugar; just deep, velvety, savory, and satisfying essence of chicken. It filled my mouth with flavor. I had the impression that the flavor reached all the way up to my temples: creating the same light-headed feeling that prolonged laughter induces.

"Fuck me dead!" I said, as I often do when a chef's creation leaves me almost speechless with pleasure.

"Yeah, Pops!!" Lucy affirmed.

No seasoning, no balancing, no fine-tuning, and yet flavor that could not have been fuller. But still, I asked myself, what was that taste? It wasn't recognizable.

That night I dreamed about it. "Umami!" I said in a dream shout that awakened me. Umami: it's in so many of the foods that form the basis of my cooking. Cooked meat has umami taste; fish too. Anchovies are umami bombs. Bacon is too. So is aged cheese. Wine has umami. Tomatoes have a form of umami. True, there is not a lot of protein in tomatoes, but perhaps it's an evolutionary adaptation that makes tomatoes most palatable when their seeds are ready to germinate. In other words, since tomatoes rely on animals' consuming them in order to disperse their seeds, they develop their most attractive flavor when the fruit is mature and the seeds need to be transported.

Umami is complex, and the more it is researched, the more we find it in a variety of things that we eat. I recently spoke with Harold McGee, author of the kitchen-science classic *On Food and Cooking.* We had just finished sharing a delicious salty, oniony, collagen-rich brisket sandwich at Roberta's restaurant in Williamsburg, Brooklyn. Harold told me that he had read that wine has umami, but a different kind from meat umami. This might explain why when served with food it has such a multiplier effect: combining ingredients that contain different types of umami increases flavor exponentially. Scientists call this phenomenon "synergistic umami." Thus, if you ever wondered why a cheeseburger with ketchup tastes so much better than grilled chopped meat, a slice of cheese, or ketchup eaten separately . . . think umami.

I began to see many of my favorite foods in a different and prettier light: with an amber glow, like the color of the chicken sauce. A BLT has umami in the bacon, the tomatoes, even the toast. Spaghetti and meatballs with marinara and grated Parmesan cheese has umami in the browned meat, the sauce, and the cheese. When the Japanese discovered umami they chose their word for "yummy" to describe it. Who doesn't like yummy?

BITTER

There is still one more taste that the palate discerns, but its effect is different. Where the other primary mouth-tastes work well in combination, bitter stands apart. It stops the experience of taste. The standard scientific explanation for bitter is that it is a warning signal to help us avoid harmful, even poisonous foods.

If this were all that bitter taste did, then any reasonable person would avoid it. But coffee, chocolate, red wine, arugula, almonds, cranberries, wasabi, and beer all have a bitter component, and they will not kill you. So, though it is true that we may have evolved the ability to taste bitter in order to warn us away from foods that can sicken or kill us, it is also true that, in the right proportion, bitter- or sharp-tasting foods can add to taste by keeping the palate fresh. If you eat something really rich—say, a braised short rib of beef—your palate is drowned in flavor. The bitterness in red wine or beer cleans the palate, pushes the reset button on the taste experience and, in so doing, readies you for the next delicious mouthful. Without a touch of bitterness to resensitize your palate, it becomes dulled, and each successive mouthful brings less and less of a flavor reward.

Celery is mildly bitter, which is why it goes so well with carrots and onions in the classic *mirepoix,* the first step in many French recipes—it complements the sweetness that develops in the onions and carrots. It surprised me that many Cajuns of western Louisiana, who are, after all, people of French descent, avoid celery (although they often break the rules).

I once asked a group of cooking Cajuns to explain their celery aversion. We were in a tin-roofed outbuilding at Rodney Mayeux's fire prevention business in Opelousas, about 120 miles west of New Orleans, near the city of Lafayette. The occasion was a weekly gathering of hunting and fishing buddies who cooked, made music, and talked about the next weekend's hunting and fishing. The meal began with crawfish, washed down with a long-necked Bud. Like everything else I ate in Louisiana, the crawfish were highly seasoned, with a combination of red, white, and black pepper.

Dinner continued with red beans, rice and sausage, and a hearty chicken fricassee (the Cajuns pronounce it "free-ka-SAY") prepared by Raphael Trosclair, a retired employee of the local school system. When I asked for the recipe, he told me that he began with half a bell pepper and an onion. But I knew that—everything in Cajun country starts with bell pepper and onion. Then garlic, chicken, water, red, white, and black pepper, and a roux. As an aside, Trosclair allowed that *some* people put celery in their fricassee but that he (and, by implication, anyone whose cooking he might respect) *most definitely would not.*

"Why?" I asked. I had never heard anyone express much of an

opinion about celery before. I had always thought of it as a rather unobtrusive vegetable, especially in the context of the Cajun addiction to thermonuclear amounts of cayenne and hot sauce.

"It's more Creole rather than Cajun." Cajuns believe that New Orleans cooking, with its mix of African, French, and Spanish, is more properly known as Creole. Cajun—at least according to the Cajuns—is putatively a pure descendent of the French culinary tradition.

"Celery takes over the flavor," someone else added while dumping a ladleful of cayenne into a stew pot.

The explanation that stayed with me was "It blands it up," to which I still say, "Huh?"

Blanding something up makes about as much sense as, say, de-saltifying. I think what my Cajun friend meant is that the mild bitterness of celery, which is so effective in recipes without powerful flavors, contributes very little to the kinds of recipes the Cajuns cook. The real reason, I suspect, is that if an ingredient contributes nothing then it's worth skipping. In cooking, as in most creative endeavors, less is often more. If it doesn't add FPC, then it might as well not be there.

Aroma

Often our first encounter with any food is its aroma. In the words of the French godfather of food writing, Anthelme Brillat-Savarin (1755–1826), "Smell and taste form a single sense, of which the mouth is the laboratory and the nose is the chimney; or to speak more exactly, of which one serves for the tasting of actual bodies and the other for the savoring of their gases."

Anyone who has smelled the appetizing aroma wafting off a platter of cooked food as it is brought to the table knows that smell precedes tastes. Once food is in the mouth, its aroma complements the basic tastes and adds pleasing complexity to the experience.

BULBY

Herbs and spices spring to mind when I think of ingredients that affect us through aroma, although they also directly affect the palate. Surprisingly, or at least it surprised Gray and me when we began to analyze flavor, perhaps the most important of the aromatic ingredients is neither an herb nor a spice; it is the onion, followed closely by its bulby cousins garlic, leeks, chives, and shallots. In their raw state, these vegetables are sharp and acrid, but cooking completely transforms them. They tend to broaden the overall flavor of a recipe and to accent sweetness without being sugary. I come from a long line of onion lovers and agree with my mother and my aunt Lorraine that, without onions, cuisine is unimaginable.

FLORAL HERBAL

More evanescent in their effect than the onion family, yet at times no less assertive, are the ingredients we called "floral herbal." When added to a recipe at the last minute, such herbs as basil, rosemary, tarragon, parsley, and cilantro send forth tantalizing perfumes. A sprig of rosemary placed on a pork chop, steak, or veal chop just off the grill heralds the imminent arrival of delicious food. Because these herbs contain volatile oils (i.e., they evaporate), just a little heat causes them to disperse their aromas. Used in this way, herbs set the stage and then exit. When introduced earlier in the cooking process, they have a subtler effect. Herbs with a licorice taste, such as tarragon and basil, will bring out sweet flavors. Rosemary, thyme, and oregano accent savory elements, particularly in the presence of concentrated umami. Cilantro is a natural partner to spicy chili-pepper heat.

The effect of floral-herbal ingredients is not confined to leafy green herbs. Lemon zest and ginger underscore the elements in fruits that set them apart from refined cane sugar. Olive oil is slightly floral and works well with herbs, particularly in salads or on cooked vegetables. Likewise, honey is both floral and sweet, as distinct from the less complicated sweetness of cane sugar or the nuttiness of maple syrup.

SPICED AROMATIC

Cinnamon, cloves, allspice, mace, coriander seed, cumin, saffron, cardamom, and star anise: in terms of taste on the tongue, they don't contribute very much; what taste they have is usually bitter. Like leafy green herbs, aromatic spices are often used because of their bouquet. Where herbs tend to broaden flavors, aromatic spices focus them. Cinnamon and allspice complement the sweetness in cookies. Curry powder, which is a combination of a variety of aromatic spices, will bring out the subtlety of shellfish or the depth of lamb, pork, and chicken. Black pepper, apart from its spicy heat, also highlights the fleshy, organic essence of meat.

Aromatic spices used in a rub on barbecued spareribs or a roast pork loin will get your mouth watering in advance of your first bite, but those same spices cooked in a braising liquid will infuse the finished dish with subtler notes. Although combinations of spices can transform food from merely good to really great, don't confuse adding lots of spices with being a gourmet chef. There are more combinations that don't work out than there are ones that do. My guiding principle, like the Cajuns with celery: if it doesn't add, then it detracts.

FUNKY

Finally, there is a very important highly aromatic flavor that we called "funky." It includes aged hams, cheeses, anchovies, and Thai fish sauce. Scallops are funky. So is beef—when grass-fed *and* aged, even more so. For a time, Gray and I considered using the word "stinky" rather than "funky," but feared some people might not find that an appetizing word, although we both did. Funk is what distinguishes the nuanced flavors of long-aged ham from freshly killed pork. I've never been able to put my finger on the explanation for it, but there is a unique, seductive, and overripe "cheesy" smell that characterizes Pinot Noir from the Côte d'Or. I think it may, in part, be umami, but why Pinot Noir grapes from just a few dozen miles of the northern slope of that one valley? As the theologian often answers the unanswerable: "It's a mystery."

There is something animalistically sensual, even sexy, in funky food. In many cases, such foods are in the process of fermentation and decay. As Harold McGee wrote: "Rotten grapes (wine), moldy milk (cheese) and ripened meat (ham) make our lives much more interesting." You might think that decay and rotting are the opposite of what you want in food, but, looked at from another point of view, controlled corruption—which is at the heart of the wine/cheese/ham-maker's craft—is nothing more than the breakdown of organic substances into other organic substances. By that measure, decay does through a natural chemical process what cuisine accomplishes through heat: transforming animal and plant matter into more flavorful and easily digestible components.

Funk is a flavor that works almost exclusively in savory dishes. The principal exception I have come across was the dessert course served at a clean-out-the-larder meal that David Rosengarten hosted to mark the end of truffle season. In Gascony, where truly great black truffles are harvested, if you haven't used your fresh truffles by March 15, you must can them. They grow spongy and lose flavor very quickly.

David, whose *Rosengarten Report* is one of the most informed and entertaining newsletters dealing with food, invited two Gascon chefs, Sylvain Portay and Laurent Manrique, to turn out a rustic meal, cooked in the fireplace.

Bear in mind, although we associate truffles with pricey fine dining, they are a traditional wild food in Southern Europe, and if you know what you are doing they can be gathered for free. If you go back a few hundred years, before the invention of modern restaurant dining, you will find that truffles were just a seasonal, nonluxury local item, like ramps or morels.

Although it was a raw, wintry evening, no sooner had I entered David's apartment than I began to swelter in the heat and truffle-laced smoke from the fireplace. In the hearth, two chickens hung suspended on lengths of string. Thick slices of truffle were stuffed under the skin, and a metal pan collected the smoky, truffled fat that dripped off the roasting birds, which the chef used to baste the chicken skin.

The savory courses began with quail and truffles, then a *garbure:* Gascon bean-and-cabbage soup with duck-leg confit and heaps of chopped roasted truffles. Then the perfectly roasted chicken. Next, arugula salad with chopped truffles, after which we adjourned to the den for dessert: a half-quince poached in port with truffles. It was served in a small bowl, the hollow center of each quince half filled with creamy mascarpone cheese topped with port syrup and the poached truffles, lightly chopped.

It was sweet, syrupy, smooth, crunchy, creamy, fruity, and as funky-tasting as a ripe durian on a hot, humid day. If pressed to choose, I would say it was the single most spectacular dessert I have ever eaten. *Mirabile dictu,* it required none of the precision of the baker's art that has always bedeviled my dessert-making.

Apart from that one dessert, though, I can't think of another sweet recipe where funky and sweet marry well. Oh yes, there was a slice of warm apple pie that I ate in a café in Hailey, Idaho (birthplace of Ezra Pound). It came with melted blue cheese on top. Awfully nice with a mug of fresh brewed coffee and sweet cream.

Texture

The first quality that comes to mind when you hear the word "pasta" is its smooth and slippery texture. Similarly, the most memorable characteristic of potato chips is not taste but crispness. The crust on fried chicken, the little nuggets of chocolate chips or nuts in a scoop of ice cream, the smooth creaminess of a pudding: all of these textures help us to make sense of taste. Texture is a critical part of tasting, but it is not taste and it has no flavor.

Just as the dimming of lights in a movie theater cues us that the show is about to start, texture sends out an invitation: "Get ready for a new flavor." Before we decide how a particular food tastes, we seek out its texture. Texture is a physical aspect of food, not a chemical one, and the explanation of its role in a taste narrative is mechanical. Though it is true that when food hits your palate you begin to react to primary flavors, it is only when your teeth come together and you breathe out through your nose that you experience the full flavor of food.

Among the various textures of food, crunch has primacy in triggering us to begin to engage fully in tasting. If there is no crunch, then, before we begin to evaluate a particular food, we seek out the tooth resistance found in flesh (meat, poultry, or seafood), or al-dente pasta, or risotto. With braised meats there is no crunchy crust, but through long simmering in the braising liquid, there is flavorful muscle fiber. The moment of truth arrives when your teeth cut through the meat and you exhale. All the tastes and aromas mix, and at that point you experience the full flavor of the meat. In the absence of crunch or tooth resistance, we look for the smooth, creamy consistency that one finds in ice cream, or custard, or polenta.

Why do we withhold a flavor judgment until we have gauged the texture of food? It gets back to the notion of flavor as a system of sensory shorthand: a way to choose nutritious food and to sort out worthless, even harmful food choices. Perhaps we read the crunchiness of the crust of cooked meat or bread as a signal for protein. Crispness in an apple or a leaf of lettuce denotes vitamins, freshness, and fiber. Creaminess can signify digestibility and ripeness.

Hunger propels us to seek food. Taste, aroma, and texture simplify our search. If you understand flavor, and if, whenever you shop, eat, or cook, you think about how to maximize its pleasures without simply resorting to sugar, salt, and fat, then, even if you have never heard the term, you understand Culinary Intelligence.

CHAPTER V The Joy of Cooking

You can read every diet book in the store. You can shop locally, seasonally, sustainably. You can count calories and avoid franchises. But only cooking leaves you fully in charge of what you eat and how it is prepared. It is the surest way to put Culinary Intelligence into practice.

Is it possible to eat a healthy and satisfying diet without cooking? Probably, but I am not the best person to tell you how. I have always cooked: from my early jobs as a summer-camp burger flipper to after-school soda jerk, to steamer of pastrami, corned beef, and knishes, to cook-in-residence on a hippie farm, and through all the years since.

Cooking is *not* about tossing lots of flaming ingredients, nor is it racing against the clock under the gaze of overcaffeinated commentators. It's not creating towering food-as-architecture. It is not a matter of using as many exotic ingredients as you can find. As Thomas Keller once told me, "Cooking is a simple equation—it's about ingredients and technique, and that's it. If it's hard, you're probably doing something wrong, because cooking is not hard; it really isn't."

Cooking, at its most basic level, is the art of adding just the right amount of heat to ingredients. It takes tough and bitter artichokes and makes them tender and nutty. Cooking transforms fibrous eggplant into a sweet mouthful that matches with the brightness of long-cooked tomatoes, the brininess of olives, the bracing aroma of rosemary. Cooking takes raw, unappetizing eggs and transmutes them into the smooth and rich foundation of an endless variety of meals. Cooking allows us to combine the fermented juice of Pinot Noir grapes (Burgundy), the flesh of a chicken, smoked salted pork (bacon), and sharp baby onions to produce the classic coq au vin. Try some of these ingredients in their uncooked state and they will be unpleasant, if not downright inedible.

Judith Jones, the visionary editor who brought the work of Julia Child, Marcella Hazan, and Madhur Jaffrey to an American public that was eager to discover the pleasures of the table, is a lifelong home cook. "I couldn't imagine feeling really alive if I weren't cooking," she told me over lunch at Molyvos, a Greek restaurant in midtown Manhattan. She had ordered grilled octopus salad, dressed with fresh herbs and lemon juice, the kind of light meal that sends food writers, their editors, and their agents back onto the hot sidewalks of New York feeling gastronomically moral.

"I so enjoyed cooking with Evan [her husband of forty-five years, who died in 1996], even though men tend to get a little bossy in the kitchen," she said with Yankee insouciance. "When I suddenly found myself living alone, I really wondered if I would continue to cook. But the alternative is worse. You walk into the apartment and the first thing you do is start something going, smelling good. It gives you warmth and anticipation. Even when you are cooking for yourself, there is a little drama and anticipation to it. In modern times, people look at cooking as something to get over with. I think we've lost something in the process. It's all rush, rush."

I agree with Judith; however, many editors of cookbooks and food articles habitually treat cooking as something to be dispensed with as quickly as possible, like sex per the advice in a Victorian marriage manual. "Too many steps, too much time," they will say when I propose a long recipe. While cooking and cleaning up for hours after a day's work may not be practical every day, there are times—holidays and weekends—when intense cooking is exactly how I want to spend my day. It is a great pleasure, made doubly so by the reward of a great meal. But preparing a daily meal need not be long and laborious. Using good ingredients in simple, quick recipes best describes my normal cooking plan.

Why does cooking bring us pleasure? Just as taste is a system of sensory shorthand that helps us sort through thousands of chemical compounds in an instant, pleasure is a highly evolved complex of emotions that tells us we are doing something that will enhance our species' chances of hanging on for another generation. In species terms, if it is pleasing, it is good: Darwin 101.

How do I know that cooking is a pleasure? Because I don't notice the passage of time when I cook. I feel the same way about my other great passion, fly-fishing. With a chef's knife (or a fly rod) in my hand, I am always in the moment. There is nothing I would rather be doing. There is nothing else that I think about. The irksome concerns of daily life are, for the most part, banished. In the "real world"—that is to say, the world outside of cooking and fishing—a task of minutes can weigh like empty hours; but a day spent in the kitchen (or on the stream) passes in a moment. But what a full moment! I truly believe that the only people who don't take pleasure in cooking are those who don't yet know how to cook. It is never too late to learn. It's in our nature.

Again, this is not an argument in favor of long recipes. If a recipe is complicated and time-consuming and it produces a great result, I'm all for it. If it's long and not so great, I'll pass. The most important thing in any recipe is that it should be the simplest route to the desired outcome. It should only be as long and complicated as it needs to be in order to produce maximum flavor and satisfaction: Occam's razor, imported into the kitchen. In practice, this can mean many ingredients and many steps, or very few ingredients and a quick, simple process.

I experienced this contrast vividly while researching a show that I produced for the Food Network in Oaxaca, Mexico. A number of sources had told me that I needed to visit a fantastic home chef, Emilia Arroyo.

We met in her sunny walled garden on a hillside in the Volcanes neighborhood of Oaxaca City: a riot of lemon and grapefruit trees, rosebushes, and climbing bougainvillea framed a wood oven and grill. Emilia and I sat in the sun—warm enough to feel good but not too hot. We chatted for a while, falling into easy conversation like friends who had not seen each other for years but who pick up where they left off. I quickly learned that her husband, a prominent judge, had died a few years before. In her grief, Emilia left her job as chief administrator of nurses in the local medical district.

"I was depressed. I couldn't do anything," she said, "so I went up to the mountains to a *curandero* [a shaman or medicine man]. I stayed with him for six months. People with all kinds of afflictions—both physical and spiritual—came to his home, hoping that he could cure them. He and his wife taught me how to cook dishes with wildflowers and mountain herbs. With time, I felt better. I returned to the city and began to cook and teach in my garden."

"Do you think it would be possible to meet this *curandero?*" I asked, fully expecting that he lived in a very remote place and rarely received any visitors, and when he did, they first had to endure an eight-day prayer vigil in light clothing on a chilly mountaintop.

To my surprise, Emilia said, "Sure, let's take a cab and go right now. We'll be there in two hours. He'll see us."

I went out to the street, flagged down a cab, and off we went to Ixtlán. When we entered the village, Emilia directed the driver up a hill that overlooked the main square. "There are wild herbs up and down the mountain," she observed. We could smell them.

We pulled up to the entry of a house built into the mouth of a cave. Supplicants clustered around it: some on crutches, some missing a limb, some whose ailments were not visible but whose faces were etched with pain.

"Follow me," Emilia said, and walked straight into the cave where the holy man, Prisciliano Morales, sat in front of a fire alongside his wife, Petronila. I told them that I was interested in home cooking, not fancy restaurant dishes, and that Emilia had recommended their food.

That was Petronila's cue to offer us her *sopa de guias,* a very nuanced recipe that calls for the leaves, vines, flowers, and fruit of a zucchini-like summer squash. Two mountain herbs, *chepil* and *chepiche,* plus some salt, were the only seasoning. A piece of *elote*—i.e., a mature ear of corn—was placed in each bowl.

As for the main ingredient, the flavor of each part of the

squash presented a different and delicate variation on a single taste theme. I thought of it as a conjugation of squash. The herbs provided a bright counterpoint. The corn was a sweet chaser. All in all, a very simple recipe: four different parts of one plant, two herbs, salt, water, and an ear of corn. Had you added anything else, the elegant flavors of the squash would have been lost.

Such simplicity is one hallmark of Oaxacan cuisine. We also tasted it in Petronila's next recipe: tamales made with traditional *masa* (cornmeal and lard), wrapped in an avocado leaf, and then further wrapped and steamed in a corn husk. The avocado leaf contributed a bright spearmint note—so light that even a sprig of parsley would have masked it. Left on its own, though, it lightened and focused the broad flavor of *masa.* Those two dishes—the soup and the tamales—are examples of very spare yet complete recipes, the fullest expression of the flavors in their ingredients.

At the other end of the complexity spectrum is the crowning glory of Oaxacan cuisine, the *mole negro.* My family and I learned to prepare it ourselves, under the tutelage of Susanna Trilling, an American expatriate who teaches the Oaxacan culinary tradition at her small ranch in Etla, a few miles outside of Oaxaca City. Although the *mole negro* is famous for its inclusion of chocolate, there is much more going on in this recipe. It calls for a half-dozen peppers to be roasted, peeled, and puréed. Other ingredients include a half-dozen herbs and an equal number of spices. Furthermore, five or six kinds of nuts and seeds are ground into a paste on a *metate.* Thirty ingredients in all, and each of them requiring its own special preparation.

It takes the better part of a day to make this sauce. When you pour it over chicken or turkey, you experience layer upon layer of taste: hot and spicy, aromatic, full of umami, herbaceous.

Every note rings through, a sure sign that nothing is superfluous, so that, even though it is very complex, it too is as simple as it can be.

But there are simple two-hundred-calorie recipes and simple two-thousand-calorie recipes. My goal is flavors, combinations of ingredients and textures that satisfy and don't leave me digging into a plate overfilled with highly caloric food that I devour down to the last twirl of spaghetti. Anytime you can get more pleasure and satisfaction from fewer bites, you are heading in the right direction: FPC.

You are much more likely to achieve this goal if you cook with flavorful ingredients. Developing the most flavor with those ingredients is the task of the cook. In restaurants, fast-food establishments, and take-out businesses, too often the default is to pile on salt, sugar, fat, and crispy breadings. As anyone who has ever worked on the line in a restaurant will tell you, if you want to improve flavor in a hurry, add lots and lots of butter.

You can often tell if someone really understands cooking by watching him or her perform a repetitive task. Good cooking, like playing an instrument, requires repetition until the right way to do things becomes muscle memory. Every chef I have ever asked about cooking skills says the same thing: repetition, repetition, repetition.

I recall a scene in a camp kitchen in Africa. I was working on a story about Tanzanian food. My teacher was Hasan Iddi, a Masai tribesman, who was the chef at an exclusive safari camp serving primarily old-fashioned continental cuisine. He was pleased when I asked him to make some home-style African food.

Through the open flaps of his cook tent, we watched a small herd of impala grazing about a hundred feet from us. In the middle distance, a long file of zebras moved in convoy; the changing patterns of each zebra's coat made their stripes appear to dance in the bright sunlight. The smell of wood smoke filled the air from huge brush fires on the horizon. The massive blazes could have been ignited by the regular late-afternoon display of heat lightning, but just as likely, game poachers had set them, knowing that, with the next rain, the burnt-over land would green up and attract grazing animals: easy targets.

As he did every day, Hasan made chapattis, the flat bread that Tanzanians eat with every meal. Because of Tanzania's proximity to the Indian Ocean, the chapatti of India has, over the centuries, found its place even this far inland, among the pastoral Masai.

In an efficient but unhurried rhythm, he never varied his movements as he made a hundred chapattis: each ball of dough rolled, trimmed, then rolled up again like a croissant and, finally, flattened. It struck me, as it has while watching Gray Kunz julienne a lemon peel, that such evenly paced, consistent, precise movement is the mark of someone who takes pleasure in cooking.

Few authorities will tell you that being able to roll chapattis, dice onions, or trim green beans while in this trancelike state is essential to good cooking, but being able to lose yourself in the moment is a sure sign that cooking brings you pleasure. And if it brings you pleasure, then the chances are you will be good at it, if you are not already.

Get Down with Brown

Browning ingredients is among the best ways I know to create satisfying flavor without additional calories. It's right up there with developing umami as a way to add FPC. There are two kinds of browning, both equally appealing.

The first is caramelization—adding heat to carbohydrates. It happens, for example, when you sauté onions, leeks, celery, carrots, or garlic. The nutty and sweet flavor in the vegetables becomes deeper, sweeter, more savory. They complement every other ingredient they are cooked with. Chefs call them "aromatics" for good reason: the aromas (volatile chemicals released through caramelization) are very appealing.

Think of all the recipes that start by instructing the cook to "sauté onions until golden and translucent." It is probably the most frequent direction in cookbooks. The reason for the directive is that it works so well. When you approach a house where someone is browning onions, even before opening the door you know what's going on inside: good food. The same goes for garlic, shallots, or leeks. When heated, the sugar molecules in the vegetables break down into hundreds of flavor compounds. They produce very forward aromas that tend to fill up the thousands of receptors in your nasal passage. The indispensable *mirepoix, sofrito,* and *battuto* that are the basis of French, Spanish, and Italian cuisine are all variations on this caramelizing theme.

The second form of browning takes place when you add heat to protein-rich ingredients such as meat, fish, or poultry. The effect on flavor is similar to caramelization but profoundly deeper. The magic involved is a more complex process, known as the Maillard reaction. Browning meat, fish, and poultry à la Maillard will transform a platter of indifferent-tasting flesh into one that packs rich flavor and sublime texture. Since all living things contain some protein, even caramelized vegetables can be Maillardized to some extent.

Although I had read the occasional snippet about the Maillard reaction in food literature, I didn't begin to comprehend just what sorcery it works until I researched my book *Pig Perfect.*

In the west of Spain, the motherland of great ham and pork, I visited with Professor Jorge Ruiz at the Veterinary Faculty of the University of Extremadura in Cáceres. "Give someone a piece of raw pork, lamb, and beef," he told me, "and ask him to identify it by taste. Most people cannot tell you much more than that it is flesh. But we all can recognize the flavor of cooked meat."

One thing that draws us so powerfully to many meat recipes is the process first explained by Camille Maillard, a French physician and scientist at the turn of the last century. It is at the core of why much grilled food tastes so good, why bread has a crispy brown crust, why a T-bone steak is always better with a charred crust and forgettable without it.

Adding heat to combine the natural sugars and amino acids in food initiates a chemical process that produces a cascade of enticing flavor compounds (even more than simple caramelizing of vegetables), among them the aroma that wafts off a grilled steak or a sizzling burger.

When the process of combining proteins and sugars takes place over the course of years and the heat is supplied by the climate of summer in Andalucía, Ruiz theorized, the result of the Maillard reaction is the complex flavor of great *ibérico* ham. When you prepare a meal with higher heat over a short period of time—such as cooking on your stove or grill—the Maillard reaction takes place in a matter of minutes. Please take note: if a recipe instructs you to brown meat, don't give it a light tan. You need to create a dark-brown crust.

When Michel Richard, with whom I wrote two cookbooks, invented his much-in-demand seventy-two-hour short ribs, the Maillard reaction is what transformed this from a blah recipe to a memorable meal. Michel, who combines a puckish Santa Claus mien and the thick Gallic accent of Charles Boyer, is revered by chefs for his flawless technique and endless curiosity. He is always inventing new recipes.

Like every top chef I know, he has been captivated by *sous-vide* cooking over the last few years. The literal translation of *sous vide* is "under pressure," referring to the way that ingredients are vacuum-sealed in a plastic pouch before being submerged in a constant-temperature water bath, between 120 and 140 degrees. This technique requires costly equipment, so it may never become a mainstay of home cooking. When meat is cooked this way, even the toughest cuts eventually become quite tender as the connective tissue, or collagen, melts and hydrates the muscle fibers in unctuous gelatin. It is a high-tech, super-low-temperature way of achieving the barbecue chef's nirvana—i.e., cooking "low and slow." In addition to creating lovely texture, any inherent umami taste grows more pronounced.

Michel had the idea of preparing short ribs using the *sous-vide* method. When cooked quickly, this cut of meat is as tough as a cavalry saddle. Conventional braising produces beautifully succulent and tender meat. He guessed that if he used *sous vide* for, say, seventy-two hours, at 120 degrees, the result would be even more tender, with the rosy-red interior of a prime steak. Throw in the fact that filet mignon was going for $24 a pound and short ribs were $4.99, and Michel had a compelling argument for *sous-vide* beef.

We were working on our cookbook in his kitchen at Citronelle, his flagship Washington, D.C., restaurant, when his first try at short ribs hit the seventy-two-hour mark. By "working" I mean we had gone off on our usual dozen conversational tangents: about tomatoes and why they were not great last year, the problem with cilantro (I like it, he doesn't), the best time of day to watch pretty girls walk by Citronelle's sidewalk tables on 30th Street, the virtues of chocolate-chip cookies, which he holds to be one of America's greatest contributions to world cuisine, and what time we would smoke our daily cigars.

David Deshaies, Michel's executive chef, came to the table with a plateful of *sous-vide* short ribs.

It was ten in the morning, which was no obstacle to Michel's calling for some Côte du Rhône.

"We need to test this under battle conditions," he explained. I agreed.

We required no knives to cut the meat; it was fork-tender. Michel took a forkful. David and I did the same. Nothing special. The meat was soft and juicy, but mostly it tasted boring.

Michel closed his eyes and smacked his lips: the master in his meditative state. He looked up and, with the middle-distance gaze of a shaman emerging from a trance, he commanded, "Season it and roast it off in a very hot pan to give it a crust." For my benefit he added, "We will Maillardize!," since I had talked to him about this subject frequently.

Take two: we bit into a crunchy, well-seasoned, mouth-watering crust on the meat (the earliest culinary trick in the human repertoire, probably invented within forty-eight hours of the first use of fire). I tell you this tale of the Maillardized crust by way of saying that cuisine, even something as simple as crusting a piece of meat, is a transformative process. By doing this, Michel added the final touch that created overall flavor of such power and intensity that just a few slices, and not a plateful, was stimulating and satisfying.*

**Historical Presidential-Trivia Footnote:* President Obama and his wife went on a dinner date to Citronelle shortly after his inauguration. The President ordered, and finished, the seventy-two-hour short ribs.

Cooking with Imagination

Every chef I have known spends a lot of time dreaming up recipes. Every good home cook has the same kind of culinary reveries. Just as a composer hears melodies in his mind before committing them to paper, cooks taste recipes before they put pan to fire.

And then they go to the market.

Next, almost without fail, serendipity strikes, leading in different, surprising, and wonderful directions.

Perhaps a recipe in a book stirs my interest, or I smell some Moroccan spices from a street-corner falafel stand, or I was reading a mystery novel the night before and mentions of a plate of freshly grilled sardines and a Portuguese Vinho Verde lodged in my memory. Once I am thus stimulated, a food daydream takes me away, and I smell, see, and even taste a fantasy. Here, for example, is the story of a waking food dream I had this spring and the meal it produced. It took shape as I was looking over an old story I had written about a great country ham that I first came across at Newsom's Old Mill Store in Princeton, Kentucky.

I envisage the ham house of Nancy Newsom, filled with four thousand mold-encrusted country hams whose funky smell fills the humid old barn with the perfume of smoky aging meat.

Cut to:

A visit to a bourbon distillery near Lexington that draws its water from a limestone stream. Limestone creates the bluish cast in bluegrass that is said to explain why the elegant leg bones of Thoroughbred horses raised in Kentucky are so strong. Chestnut horses, their coats iridescent in the sunlight, dissolve into the image of another product that originated in Kentucky that floats across my inner field of vision: Bibb lettuce—lacy, crisp, and as crinkly as rime ice.

Okay: I have the beginning of an idea for dinner. I leave my desk. It's two-thirty in the afternoon. No sooner do I step into Jim & Andy's, the greengrocer around the corner from my house, than a shipping carton full of bright-green broccoli rabe catches my eye, as Carmine Cincotta no doubt intended. I ask for his opinion. He knows that I am interested in great, not just good. He lifts his pencil from his ever-present *New York Times* crossword puzzle and, with a "trust me" tilt of his eyebrows, tells me, "The restaurants have all been buying it and I had some left over. It's really good."

I cross Bibb lettuce off the shopping list and stroll down a new avenue of food fantasy. My newly purchased broccoli rabe is a new jumping-off point for a dinner recipe. "Clams," I tell myself. "It wants clams."

So I cross Court Street and buy a dozen littlenecks at my local seafood store, Fish Tales. The meal is taking shape.

I envisage sautéing the broccoli rabe quickly, maybe tossing in some red-pepper flakes. I'll serve it over a few ounces of penne cooked in clam broth. Common culinary wisdom has it that you don't ever serve cheese with shellfish, but in my imagination I can clearly taste peppery, funky, deeply savory grated pecorino. To hell with conventional wisdom.

Hmm . . . something's missing. I close my eyes and go through the motions of tasting, smacking my lips together, hoping that this response will summon a delicious taste memory. "Got it!" I need a half-pound of a thin sausage—made with a mixture of pork, spices, broccoli rabe, and mozzarella. It is sold farther down Court Street, at Esposito's pork store. Such stores, which are often found in old Italian neighborhoods, make their own sausages and sell all cuts of pork. They also sell fresh pasta, cheeses, and seemingly every brand of canned tomato ever canned. The sausage is curled around on itself, impaled on two sharpened dowels set at ninety-degree angles, so that it looks like a pinwheel.

I remember the last time I had this lovely sausage:

Lambeau Field in Green Bay, Wisconsin, the home of the Packers, the clearest of blue-sky days in late fall, very cold. But the bitterest cold cannot put a damper on the party outside the stadium. A number of Packer partisans sport green-and-gold body paint, their shirtless state best explained by their having grown inured to the cold, or perhaps simple inebriation.

Smoke belches from home-welded barbecue rigs that look like the scavenged machinery in Road Warrior. *The crowd, as big as an army encampment, stretches as far as I can see in all directions. Dueling rock anthems blast out of makeshift stereos. Burly bikers, beach chairs, bratwurst, and beer.*

Like a gold nugget glinting amid the bratwurst, taco salads, and venison chili, a familiar though unexpected pinwheel-sausage shape stops me in my tracks.

"Hey, what's that sausage?" I ask the group gathered around the grill.

"Don't know what it's called. My brother sent it from an Italian store in Brooklyn."

"Not Esposito's?" I say, with a what-a-small-world inflection.

"You know—that's what it said on the bag."

The die is cast. I walk a half-mile to Carroll Gardens and into Esposito's, buy the sausage, make the recipe. Really good. Just what I wanted.

I find such dreams and fantasies indispensable to eating well and intelligently. As in dreams, one image sometimes shifts, seemingly without reason, to another. Go with it. Your appetite is telling you something. It opens up new choices. Every time you shop, every time you stand at the stove, every time you mull over your choices on a menu, you make taste choices. We live in a food environment that always presents the option of an industrially processed quick fix—something sweet and creamy or salty and fatty, or all four at once. You can bolt it down in a hurry and then get on with your day.

Don't. Instead, devote some thought to what tastes you want to experience, in what order, and in what amounts, and thereby begin a process that culminates in sitting down to a meal and enjoying every bite to the fullest. It's the only way I know to take control of what I eat. Have fun with it, try new ideas, let pleasure be your guide. With a little CI it will never fail you.

CHAPTER VI Breakfast, Lunch, and Dinner (and Everything In Between)

Part I: Breakfast

It is basic human nature to seek variety and new experiences, but breakfast is often an exception. People tend to treat it as a routine: predictable and much the same every day, whether it's a donut, a bagel, granola, yogurt, or fresh fruit. For that reason, there may be some truth to the well-worn adage repeated by millions of mothers since the Dawn of Eating that breakfast is the most important meal, if only because we get in the habit of having the same things each morning and thereby set a caloric benchmark for the rest of the day.

Although there are people who never eat breakfast, I need something in my belly to get my day going. Most people do.

I have an affectionate feeling toward the idea of breakfast: the morning light streaming through the window, a breeze stirring the branches of the sycamore in the backyard, birdsongs, the closing of car doors and the labored start-up of car ignitions, the brisk footfalls of earlier risers on their way to the day's activity. Even a big city feels more villagelike and less bristling with aggressive energy in these early hours. At such times, sipping a mug of hot coffee while reading the news is a grand way to transition from the realm of dreams into the world of workaday concerns.

You don't have to look your best to impress anybody at breakfast (unless you have the bad luck to have a breakfast meeting scheduled). Soon enough, you will shift into gear and the nonstop business of the day, but for ten minutes, twenty minutes—whatever you can spare—breakfast is as close to a meditation moment as many of us are likely to get. Clearly, this idyllic picture doesn't apply to the bedlam in a house when children need to be roused, fed, and sent off to school. (Unless you get up before the kids do.)

You are in a psychological comfort zone and therein lies the danger. You feel laid-back, relaxed; no one is looking over your shoulder. So, while you are still in the nonjudgmental home environment, you warm up a four-hundred-calorie muffin, or eat two and a half slices of French toast (you intended only one for yourself, but the kids left some behind). Maybe you have some leftover pie, or a Danish, or a fresh buttery croissant upon which you spread more butter and perhaps some jam. Or, in extremis, there's always a microwave ready to accommodate a slice of leftover pizza.

Bad ideas all around, which gets me back to the concept of breakfast as the most important meal. If you carb up, and throw in a lot of sugar and butter to boot, then perhaps breakfast is both the most important and the most dangerous meal: having got the day off to such a poor start, you will be playing caloric catch-up for the next sixteen to eighteen hours.

No one, in my experience, cuts back on calories as the day progresses. Mario Batali concurs. He belongs to the "What you don't eat can't make you fatter" school of breakfast. He skips breakfast. As he explained to me, "Even though my wife is fond of the old saying 'You have to have the breakfast of a king, the lunch of a prince, and the dinner of a pauper,' if I have the breakfast of a king, I have the lunch of a king—I keep going all day. Once I have my engine going, I need more. So I try to just have coffee and wait until lunch."

Sam Sifton, a fellow member of the foodoisie, was the restaurant critic of the *New York Times*. In many ways he reminds me of a younger me. He is passionate about two things, fishing and food. We also share a body type, the kind that puts weight on if we don't pay proper attention to what and how much we eat. Given the fact that Sam had all of New York as his smorgasbord, you would think that he could pick and choose what he eats in a way that mere civilians cannot. But most of his calories came in the form of restaurant food prepared by chefs who always want to blow the customer's mind with flavor, often no matter how much sugar, salt, and fat might end up on the plate.

At breakfast, Sam is in command, to the degree that his kids let him be. "I have two small children who expect a hot meal every morning," he told me. "That includes steel-cut oatmeal, or organic cream of wheat, and fresh fruit. Once every ten days or so, I like an egg sandwich."

This is an example of the benefits of a child-driven breakfast strategy. In choosing what to feed our children, we tend to step back from "What do I feel like having right now?" Instead, we are more likely to think about CI when we are looking after the health of our children. Whole grains, whole fruit, and eggs are terrific choices for kids. They also make for a fine breakfast for the rest of us. "Doing it for the children" is a larger CI principle that can be extended beyond breakfast. Before you make up your mind about what to eat at any meal, ask yourself, "Would I want my children to eat this?"

With my breakfasts, as with Sam's, steel-cut oatmeal is in heavy rotation on the list. It is made of whole kernels of oats that are cut into a few pieces. This means it is virtually unprocessed. Served with whole-milk yogurt from the farmers' market, a few cut-up prunes, and a drizzle of maple syrup, it is completely satisfying and delicious. Rolled oats are okay, but they usually have the outer bran removed, and that means they are somewhat processed and more quickly absorbed and turned into sugar. Instant or quick-cooking oats are even more processed and, therefore, farther down my list of healthy choices. The CI principle here is, the closer a cereal product is to the piece of grain that came off the stalk, the more highly I recommend it. This applies to any breakfast cereal, hot or cold. The mouth-feel of steel-cut oatmeal is comforting, smooth in texture with bite-worthy nuggets that are mildly nutty in flavor. I could eat it every day, if not for the fact that it takes a half-hour to cook and you have to stir the pot from time to time.

It was nice to see eggs among Sam's options. Somewhere in the last twenty years or so, the diet geniuses found the Secret to Eternal Life: *don't eat eggs!* Such hysterical edicts remind me of humorist Redd Foxx's comments about health foods and fads: "All these people are trying to be healthy: stopping smoking, drinking, eating chicken necks. They're going to feel like damn fools when they're lyin' in their hospital beds dyin' of nothin'."

The cholesterol issue is not uncomplicated, but remember that cholesterol is not a chemical additive invented by big food conglomerates to adulterate our food. The brain needs cholesterol. Without it, we would have the same mental wattage as a plant. Eggs are packed with nutrition, and nature has designed such an aesthetically pleasing package for them that I find it hard to believe that a sublime food, which humans have always eaten, became a virtual poison in the last thirty years. Farm fresh eggs with the deep-orange yolks that come from healthy free-range chickens are nutritious and flavorful. They taste good all by themselves, require no melted cheese or other flavor enhancers beyond salt and black pepper. They do have cholesterol, but the many scientific studies indicate that most, if not all, of our cholesterol is manufactured by our bodies from other components of our diet, such as fats. Still, even if cholesterol is a concern and you want to hedge your bets (depending on which scientist you believe), there's no need to give up your eggs. I eat them about twice a week.

When I am on the road, I often forget my own advice in this regard and regularly order eggs every day. Blame it on Lord Nelson, who, in addition to being England's greatest naval hero, was also notorious for an extramarital affair that he carried on with the wife of a British diplomat in Italy. When pressed about this moral lapse he replied, "East of Gibraltar, all men are bachelors." When it comes to deciding whether to order eggs, I am one of Nelson's bachelors, and Gibraltar is in my rearview mirror. If the choice is between eggs, a bear claw, or a Krispy Kreme, I go for eggs every time.

The challenges of kick-starting the dining day on the road are usually greater than eating at home. Temptingly described breakfasts fit for a lumberjack—maybe two lumberjacks—are the norm. Consider this menu, full of cutesy names, offered at a log-cabin-style restaurant in eastern Wyoming. First, the SNOWBORDER, a pun that conflates snowboarding with "south of the border": a breakfast burrito that consisted of scrambled eggs, sautéed onions, peppers, tomatoes, cheese, and a choice of ham, bacon, or sausage, rolled in a flour tortilla and served with salsa, sour cream, and hash browns. I'm guessing, based on nutritional information I've found for similar burritos, that you're talking about a breakfast of about 950 calories. The HOMESTEADER promised a Belgian waffle, two eggs, and ham, bacon, or sausage. Right above it, by way of suggestion, there was a picture of a waffle topped with hot fudge and strawberries. The BIG BEAR featured three eggs and a choice of ham, bacon, or sausage with biscuits, country sausage gravy, and hash browns. There are so many calories here, and it's all so loaded with fat, the three eggs almost slip in under the radar.

Who, I wonder, needs or wants three eggs for breakfast? I usually have one egg. When I cook eggs at home, three eggs make two nice omelets. With so many other things dwarfing the eggs on the restaurant breakfast plate, you might need three eggs to make it look as if you are getting your money's worth in the egg department. This gets into the issue of portion size, which I'll take up later.

Everywhere I looked I saw the same words—"bacon," "sausage," "egg," "cheese," "pancake," and "waffle"—arranged in all possible permutations, like the dancing pink elephants in baby Dumbo's drunken nightmare. You could have tossed a dart at the menu and anything it hit would have been equally loaded with calories. I chose the à-la-carte route, ordering a poached egg on rye toast with crisp bacon on the side. Why bacon? Because, when you are in a room swirling with the aroma of frying pork, salt, and spices, ignoring such appetite-inducing stimuli will probably cost your body more in stress than it does in extra calories.

Closer to my daily experience is the routine of Danny Meyer, the leading New York restaurateur of the last two decades. In spite of his passion for food and wine, he has always kept pretty trim.

As he told me, "Audrey [Danny's wife] buys granolas and other whole-grain cereals from Whole Foods, and that's my breakfast at home. When I go to the gym for an eight o'clock workout, I have a protein shake after the workout. On the weekends, one day Daddy makes eggs for everybody and on the other day one of the kids will make pancakes or we have bagels."

We are looking at three common breakfast strategies here: I think of them as the Automatic Default, the Quickie, and, in the case of the above-mentioned pancakes and bagels, the Weekend Reward.

First the Automatic Default. It's something that you can reasonably enjoy every day. It's fast to make or to order. And, most important, you have it so often that you don't even have to take up precious morning bandwidth thinking about it. These days, my go-to breakfast is similar to Dan's: whole-grain cereal with almonds, fresh blueberries (or dried cranberries), and milk (I prefer whole milk for its flavor). Almonds have healthy fats and protein; berries add some sweetness and are high in antioxidants; the cereal has high-fiber complex carbohydrates that are not converted instantaneously into sugar and is pleasantly crunchy; the milk adds protein, flavor, and moistness. Granolas, though they are touted to be healthful, are usually quite high in sugar. True, they are good sources of fiber, and there are nutrients in their dried fruit, but the calories count. Better to add some dried fruit, for flavor and texture, to a less sweet whole-grain cereal than to eat four to five hundred calories of granola (forget about the suggested serving size on the box and consider how much a real person puts in a bowl).

Many "healthy" breakfast cereals appeal to our historical sense with a line or two on the box about how ancient and nutritious the grains are. No matter what the label says, don't for a minute think that the Babylonians or ancient Romans ate multigrain flakes. Breakfast cereals (flakes and nuggets) are a new class of food, invented in America at the end of the nineteenth century, when huge grain surpluses mounted as a result of the enormous harvests that piled up to feed more livestock. Two nineteenth-century food pioneers and health-food nuts—W. K. Kellogg and C. W. Post—came up with dried cereals as a way to sell this surplus in the form of whole-grain breakfast cereals.

So far, no CI problem.

It was only when these products began to include increasing amounts of sugar and other additives that they became a dietary liability. Still, there are plenty of healthful breakfast cereals that satisfy me in the morning and keep hunger at bay until lunchtime. In choosing one, I always look at the ingredient list to confirm that whole grains are at the head of the list and that there's not a lot of stealth sugar wheedling its way in under a variety of aliases.

As for the Quickie—the protein shake—I am not a believer but I'm not anti. In reply to an e-mail on the subject of protein shakes, NYU professor and leading expert on nutrition Marion Nestle wrote to me, "They are the illusion of food." It's not that protein shakes are bad for you, or that some aren't better than others. It's just that I have an inherent distrust of deconstructed foods—whether they are Slim-Fasts or much more organic custom mixes. They are, by definition, collections of nutrients, so they do not promote a whole-food mind-set. My choice here is a nutritious smoothie made from plain yogurt, a frozen banana, fruit (berries, mangoes, peaches), and whole milk. You may have seen kefir in the store. It's another fermented milk product, like buttermilk or thin yogurt. Perfect in a smoothie, no added milk needed.

Before Danny settled on his current default breakfast, his pre-CI version was built around the bagel. On the plus side, you can find bagels everywhere, and, even more important for someone interested in getting breakfast out of the way without a fuss, you can eat them anywhere: walking on the street, cradling your phone in one ear, riding in a car, pushing a baby stroller, or standing on a bus or subway, sitting on an airplane. As with pizza, you can put almost anything on a bagel: among others, poppy seeds, onion flakes, salt, dried garlic, onions, cheddar cheese in any combination.

"In the old days, before I started going to the gym," Danny said, "I would drop my daughter off at school. I'd go straight to the bagel store on Eighty-sixth Street and get a poppy-seed bagel with cream cheese. Then I'd go one block west to Papaya King and get fresh-squeezed orange juice. Finally, I would take my bagel and OJ to the Starbucks on Lex and Eighty-seventh, and I would order coffee and I would sit in the window—this is before the days when I had a BlackBerry. I would read the newspaper with my bagel and OJ and coffee, and that's how my day would start.

"I had no idea at that time that bagels weren't very healthy, and high in calories. I didn't understand the role of carbs—that's something I really learned at the gym, from my trainer. He doesn't even believe in drinking OJ because of how high it is in sugar and carbs. So I would say that today I probably have a bagel once every two weeks, and probably a glass of OJ once a month."

On the question of orange juice, as I said before, I believe that whole fruits are better than juice, because the sugar is less slowly absorbed. If you don't want to do without your morning OJ, the kind with more pulp is preferable: slower sugar absorption.

Like Dan, I have eaten my share of bagels; and, like Dan, I have virtually—but not completely—given them up. But it wasn't processed white flour that discouraged me so much as the fact that once bagels entered mainstream food culture it became impossible to find traditional thin bagels with their lovely chewy crust. The old-time bagel has been replaced by bloated, puffy things akin to hamburger buns with a hole in the middle. People who haven't lived through the pervasive degradation of the bagel don't know what they are missing.

Giving up bagels need not mean having to forgo smoked salmon—or lox, as it was always known in my childhood. It is an excellent food: high in heart-healthy fat and not particularly caloric. Even in a bagel-free environment it's terrific on toast with a very light shmear, which is Newyorkspeak for a coating of cream cheese. Or, if no cream cheese, a little butter. The fat in the butter melts and moistens the dryness of the bread to more nearly match the succulence of the salmon. The bread should be whole-grain and full-flavored, which is the kind the Scandinavians eat their smoked salmon with.

Finding good smoked salmon, though not so difficult as finding a good bagel, is not as easy as it was in the days when many neighborhoods in the New York area had what was called an "appetizing store" that sold lox, smoked whitefish, sturgeon, chopped liver, pickled herring, Austrian hard candies (with soft jam-filled centers), raspberry-flavored marshmallow twists, nuts, and dried fruits. The mix of aromas was intense, complex, and unforgettable, in the way that childhood sense memories remain evocative and stimulating for the rest of your life.

There was always one guy who was the A-level lox slicer. You would peer through the glass case as he worked, making sure he didn't include too much of the gray meat in the very middle and, above all, that he never sliced the salmon very thickly. It was said of a good knife man that if he did his job well one could read the *New York Times* through one of his slices.

Those places do not exist anymore; nor, so far as I have been able to see, does lox made from wild Atlantic salmon. When you see smoked salmon advertised as "Scottish" or "Irish," all that means is that it came from a fish farm in one of those countries. For the most part, the taste of farmed salmon is the same no matter where it comes from. If you want wild—which in my book has better flavor—get packaged salmon from Washington State, British Columbia, or Alaska. Scientifically speaking, Pacific salmon is not true salmon, but the taste is close enough, especially when smoked and salted.

I could easily eat smoked salmon more often than I do. When I visit my parents I have it every day. It is expensive, though, so at home I think of it as something special to vary my breakfast or lunch routine. When our children were young, we'd have pancakes or French toast with real maple syrup on Saturday, and bagels with lox and pastries on Sunday. It's probably no accident that the era of bagels and pancakes marked my most dramatic weight gains.

When the kids get older, and you graduate from the Weekend Reward pancake option on Saturday, and watching your weight leads you to cut back on bagels and lox on Sunday, make sure you move on to something with high FPC. A frittata or an omelet, with sautéed diced pepper and onion lightly sprinkled with vinegar, has no processed ingredients and is low in calories, but has a huge amount of FPC. If there is some country ham or prosciutto on hand, crisp a few slices in olive oil and serve on the side. Deglaze the pan with black coffee for a low-cal version of red-eye gravy; it cleans your palate, setting you up for a fresh taste with the next bite. In season, fry some tomato halves, cut side down, until they begin to blacken, and serve alongside.

Another of our breakfasts is Melinda's superb whole-grain muffins, studded with nuts, fresh blueberries, or dried cranberries. It's also a great way to use up overripe peaches, bananas, or mangoes. They cry out for a smidge of jam, and I give in. Not a calorie-packed glob, just a tasty smidge.

You don't need pastries or coffee cake, ever. If you do have them, you may not catch up calorically until Wednesday, and that's just two days before the next weekend, and thereby starts your dietary ski-run down a perilously icy slope. If your weekend breakfasts are heavy on Flavor per Calorie, you really won't miss the sugary stuff.

For many of us, breakfast without coffee is unthinkable. A few years ago, I began to include homemade cappuccino in my morning routine, shortly after we were given a marvelous import from Italy called the Aerolatte, which foams milk without all that messy steaming (you just quickly microwave the milk, then froth it). It's not very often that you find something costing less than twenty bucks that improves your life on an everyday basis, but the Aerolatte does. It makes great foam. In fact, it was so good that I quickly upped my consumption from one mug to three, and because I used skim milk, I never gave the calories a second thought. But skim milk isn't water. Water has no calories per cup. Skim milk has ninety. In other words, nearly three hundred calories' worth of milk in the morning's coffee.

Here we have a classic dieting dodge—a phony trade-off—in which a lower-calorie substitute—in this case, skim milk—is treated as a license to consume a lot more of the substitute. The result was that the amount of skim milk I consumed was the caloric equivalent of two and a half glasses of wine at breakfast. Once I realized this, I went back to regular coffee with about an ounce of richer and sweeter whole milk to soften the coffee's bitterness and to cool it down. That's a net pickup of over two hundred calories a day, which, if you multiply those savings over the course of a year . . .

But I'm not going there. Out of such math are two-week cheeseburger binges born.

Part II: Five Ways of Looking at Lunch

One of the hallmarks of being human, though not unique to our kind, is that we treat meals as social occasions. When we eat with others, we strengthen the bonds that knit us into society. When it is time to eat, we have always come together: with family, with friends, with colleagues at work. We mark the important events in life with special meals, always shared with others. One exception to this rule, in modern America—and, increasingly, in the rest of the world—is lunch.

In our multitasked, twenty-four/seven culture, lunch has become a pit stop, a momentary detour, as necessary as a trip to the bathroom, and often as brief. After three or four hours of work, you need a bite: something quick, so that you can get back to the job.

While most people have an idea of what constitutes breakfast or what dinner looks like, lunch is more of a catch-as-catch-can meal. Is it a glorified snack, one among many in our eat-whenever-it-crosses-your-mind workday? Is it a mid-sized meal to be bolted down in ten minutes? Or is it a chance to unwind, enjoy the day, maybe close a business deal, and, in the best of all possible worlds, get ready for a nap?

Ask any five people for an example of lunch and you could easily get five different answers.

1. A sandwich or a burger, with fries
2. The salad bar
3. Fruit-flavored yogurt
4. Six oysters, a veal chop with wild mushrooms and sautéed spinach, one glass of Sancerre, two glasses of Pinot Noir, an apple tart, espresso, Armagnac, and a cigar
5. Nothing

For much of my working life, lunch was a no-brainer. I walked a block or two, and had a couple of slices of pizza. When I reformed my diet, pizza and I mutually separated. The critical point in my pizza routine had never been that second slice. It was foreordained, because I had ignored my hunger pangs until I was ravenous. "I don't care about the calories," I told myself. "Pizza is the quickest food fix I can find. Feed me now!"

It's at times like these—when hunger trumps intelligence—that high fat, lots of white flour, and high-calorie fast food don't seem so out of the question. Maybe a Burger King Double Croissan'Wich (570 calories) or Chili's Texas Cheese Fries with Chili and Jalapeño Ranch (2,070 calories!).

The time to apply CI most effectively is before, not after, you are hungry enough to eat a cheese-filled baseball mitt. Ideally, you may have already done all the culinary thinking you need the day before, and the answer may be found in your refrigerator, in the form of the often overlooked and underappreciated category known as leftovers. Even if you don't work at home, as I mostly do, brown-bagging is an option.

By way of illustration, let's take a look in my refrigerator.

Hmm . . . olives, capers, anchovies, Parmesan cheese, Greek (i.e., thick) yogurt, strawberry jam, mango chutney now approaching its third or fourth anniversary on the same shelf inside the door. In other words, my refrigerator reflects the normal mix of staples as well as the kind of odd stragglers that find their way into the recesses of all refrigerators and eventually get squatting rights. There is also a Tupperware container with last night's polenta and a stew of baby eggplants, garlic, shallots, crushed tomatoes, and hot-pepper flakes. Also about a cup of cooked spaghetti squash and, right next to it, a bone-in breast of Sunday's roast chicken, with wing attached.

It's a mistake to think of such leftovers as sloppy seconds. *Never* throw delicious leftovers out. They are often the basis of wonderful serendipitous meals. In preparing something new made from leftovers, my goal, as always, is maximum FPC. The chicken was brined in a solution of salt, honey, and bay leaves (see recipe, page 221), so, even though it was white meat, which when it reaches the leftover phase tends to dryness, it was still moist and flavorful. According to *Cook's Illustrated*—which analyzes food with actuarial precision—it's at least 7 percent moister than white meat that is not brined. This may not seem like a big deal, but it's the crucial difference between meat that is washcloth-dry and succulent, full-flavored chicken.

The leftover eggplant-tomato combo was very concentrated in flavor, an effect achieved by caramelizing the eggplant for ten minutes, then lightly browning the shallots and garlic, and baptizing it all with the one remaining glassful in a twenty-one-dollar bottle of Chablis, which, for home consumption, I rate as a not-cheap wine.

As for the spaghetti squash, Melinda had seasoned it with salt and pepper, then tossed it with olive oil, then roasted it and separated the delicious flesh from the tough skin, which was all this freshly harvested vegetable needed to bring it to its pinnacle of flavor.

On another day, my refrigerator reruns might be cold steak

with some roasted sweet peppers, or sliced leg of lamb with bacon-onion marmalade, or cooked shrimp with some extra salad greens that we washed but didn't use the night before.

You may not want to pack a sandwich or reheat your leftovers in the office microwave every day, but once or twice a week leftovers are delicious, and you will not find anything better at a restaurant or take-out place.

The general rule here is that leftovers from a meal that was thoughtfully cooked with the best ingredients will make a fine lunch (or dinner). If there was CI in the preparation of the original meal, then there will be CI in the leftovers.

For example, I can't think of a more satisfying meal than one enriched with the liquid left over from Daniel Boulud's braised short ribs (actually, he got that recipe from his grandmother Francine, whose native tongue was the ancient Romance language of Dauphinois, still spoken by a few inhabitants of the Lyon region). This rich braise usually leaves a cup or so of the richest, brawniest, winiest sauce imaginable, just the ticket for a next-day risotto made with red rice, or farro, or barley.

Oops, I almost overlooked soup. This is the culinary equivalent of forgetting a close friend's birthday: you shouldn't let it happen, but somehow it does. I love soup. So do most people, but it rarely makes it onto anybody's list of favorite foods. Why? The answer is probably no more complicated than the fact that soup isn't sexy, but when you lean over a steaming bowlful, the sensual experience is as rich and enticing as a steak or a stew. This is not surprising, because soup is usually made from whole foods: onions, carrots, fresh or leftover meat and bones, tomatoes, beans, herbs. A good soup has plenty of nutrients and often hardly any fat.

Homemade soups don't demand highly developed kitchen skills. Because they often rely on what is in your larder or the fridge, they are almost always different, and therefore rarely boring. You might not have the time or inclination to prepare your own soups, but there are many good canned soups made with real ingredients. Read the label. Packaged bean or lentil soups, which often call for the addition of fresh, whole ingredients, may seem overpriced considering the inexpensive ingredients in them, but they are nevertheless whole foods and a time-saving convenience. On a per-serving basis, they are cheap. Away from home, the soup of the day is often the best CI choice on a diner or café menu.

Even though you may have made a soup a week ago, it resists being classified as a leftover. I don't think of it as either new soup or old soup; it's simply soup, in an eternal state of having just been made. Rather than losing flavor or starting to feel tired and stale, the flavors of soup deepen during its time in the refrigerator. If, for the sake of variety, I want to change it a bit, I often reheat it with some fresh or cooked chard, kale, cabbage, or broccoli rabe and finish it with grated cheese and a drizzle of olive oil. This provides enough of a makeover to convince me that it's a new dish.

As I mentioned, when I am working at home, come lunchtime I will often open a can of sardines—in tomato sauce, mustard sauce, smoked, or salted and preserved in olive oil. Sometimes I pour the sauce over a few slices of raw onion to cut their sharpness, and save the rest of the onion for soup, an omelet, or for browning in the pan juices of a roast. It's an environmental good deed to eat little fish instead of depleting the ocean's stock of salmon, swordfish, striped bass, and other large fish from further up the food chain. But, good eco-citizenship aside, cured and smoked little fishes—a category that also includes the indispensable anchovy—also have maximum FPC and are not particularly high in calories. Granted, this lunch is not for everyone.

In America there is a cultural prejudice against "fishy"-smelling fish—mackerel, anchovies, herring. This is a shame, because it bears repeating that these are precisely the kinds of fish that are high in good-for-you omega-3's.

At the other end of the food spectrum from smelly fish is the fruit smoothie. Once or twice a week on average, I take some bananas (which we peel and freeze when they start to get overripe) and throw them in the blender with yogurt, milk, and fresh or frozen mangoes, peaches, or berries—nothing else.

When you are away from home, opening a can of sardines or making a smoothie is not very practical. Sometimes the only option is a fast-food franchise. Although menus offer many choices, basically they come down to different permutations of fat, salt, white flour, potatoes, and soft drinks. The problem is not really what to choose; it's finding *anything* that isn't made totally from processed ingredients. Many chains have added lighter eco-friendly choices, but—apart from the estimable Chipotle, known for its wholesome, sustainable food—I get the feeling that it's in the same begrudging spirit that TV networks offer equal time to third-party candidates.

A recent stop in a Taco Bell in Nebraska comes immediately to mind, but I could as easily have picked the Roy Rogers at mile sixty-five on the New York Thruway, or the Cracker Barrel near State College, Pennsylvania. Upon entering the Taco Bell, I glanced over the menu and immediately skipped everything that included melted or grated cheese, which, as in most fast-food franchises, eliminates many if not most of the menu items. Had I stopped in at a Cracker Barrel, the décor would have been different, but melted cheese would have been no less in evidence.

Whether it's on pizza, burgers, or tacos, salty, fatty melted cheese accounts for a huge amount of the calories in the American traveler's diet; menus boast cheese with more cheese and extra cheese thrown in for good measure. If they can't melt it, then they grate it or chop it and toss it on salads, pastas, or baked potatoes. In the end, all this cheese ensures that the taste of the meat or the vegetable that should be the star of the dish is drowned out. If the meat lacks flavor and texture, no matter—cheese makes up for it. This is not meant to disparage cheese. A planet without cheese is a planet I want to leave. But all cheese all the time will make even the best cheese less interesting.

As I continued to read through the menu, I was not seduced by the word "salad" and the picture of healthy-looking Chipotle Steak Taco Salad that weighed in at nine hundred calories. I thought back to the tacos I used to eat in Mexico City: some fresh salsa—usually made with tomato, chilies, onion, garlic, herbs—along with grilled meat or chicken. The closest thing to that on the Taco Bell menu was a Fresco Grilled Steak Soft Taco.

Funny, I thought, a *refresco,* at least in Mexico, means a soft drink, but I guess the word *refresco* sounds like "refreshing" in English and is probably meant to connote lightness. I opted for a couple of Taco Bell's Frescos filled with lettuce, tomato, grilled steak pieces, and salsa. On the Taco Bell Web site, the nutritional breakdown for a Fresco includes a bunch of chemicals (probably in the salsa, which you can leave on the side), but at least the principal ingredients include beef, tomatoes, and onion. If you don't eat all of the tortilla wrapping—which I rarely do—you can cut the calories nearly in half. So, although fast food is never a first choice, it is an acceptable last choice instead of, say, a bag of Cheetos or cheese-coated nachos.

Then there's always the salad option for lunch, which, especially when not freighted with a quarter-pound of blue cheese, bacon bits, and butter-soaked croutons, makes for a fine meal. Not only do fresh vegetables provide a wide range of nutrients that are not found in other foods, they fill you up. In food-science parlance, they induce satiety, so that you have less room for high-calorie food.

But salads in the through-the-looking-glass world of fast food and salad bars can be nothing more than a low-calorie come-on for formidably flavored high-calorie dressings. Flavor is good, but because so much in our food culture is predicated on our reliably choosing fat, salt, and sugar, most bottled dressings are heavy on all three, plus a lot of chemicals. So, even though you are eating salad, you are not cutting back on calories when you order a salad at McDonald's with their version of Newman's Own ranch dressing: 170 calories of salad dressing that is heavy on fat, sugar, and additives is not going to lose you any weight.

Calories are not the whole bottled-dressing story. For example, Kraft Free Ranch Fat Free Dressing, at the time of this writing, has only fifty calories per serving, but after water, the second ingredient is corn syrup and the fourth is high-fructose corn syrup (why the difference between the two sugar-rich syrups?). Then, after onion juice and garlic juice and soybean oil, you find xanthan gum, potassium sorbate, and calcium disodium, then a couple more real food derivatives, followed by disodium guanylate, disodium inosinate, spice, caramel color, and sulfiting agents. For all I know, if you left out the onion, garlic, and corn syrup, this could be the formula for a radial tire.

What almost all commercial salad dressings have in common is that they are so sweet and so thick that even the best-tasting vegetables are overwhelmed. From this, it follows that the only function the vegetables serve is texture and volume, not flavor. The logic at work here makes sense only if these ingredients have no flavor (which should be never).

Why do people bother eating salad at all in this case? Because common wisdom has it that salads are healthy. They are also a counterbalance to the rich flavors and texture of meat or fish. But when we load up something healthy with high-calorie, chemical-laden goop, it's time to face the truth, that our vegetables are taking a bath in the caloric and nutrient equivalent of Mrs. Butterworth's pancake syrup with a little vinegar thrown in.

It is far better—nutritionally, sensually, ecologically—to make salads with vegetables of the season, picked at their peak of flavor. It's also easy. You just dress with olive oil and vinegar (or lemon juice) and season with salt and pepper. Olive oil, apart from being delicious, contains no saturated fat and is very high in heart-healthy monounsaturated fat. Olive oil also helps to extract antioxidants and vitamins from plants: nutrients that would otherwise pass through your system without being utilized. In terms of flavor, vinegar or lemon juice balances the sugars in ripe fruits and vegetables and plays well against salt. You couldn't find a simpler recipe. If you add anything to this basic dressing, it might be some mashed anchovies, Dijon mustard, garlic, or finely diced shallots—all powerfully flavored whole foods.

Using simple homemade salad dressing rather than bottled or packaged commercial dressings will not only reduce the amount of calories you consume, it will also cut down on the cloying, creamy, and chemicalized flavor profile that is the hallmark of processed food. The more we eat such food, the more conditioned we become to expect it in everything we eat. Culinary Intelligence is, in part, about dialing out the marketing noise and deconditioning yourself.

You can always have fresh salad, even in the winter. For example, a salad of celery, radishes, and parsley tossed with lemon juice and olive oil is crunchy, fresh, and flavorful. Salad greens from Texas, California, and Florida, although they are not local to my area, travel reasonably well when the Midwest and the East are in a deep freeze. They won't be June or July wonderful, but with the help of a good vinaigrette, Sunbelt greens are still tasty, crisp, and filling. Dark bread, a piece of cheese, and a bit of leftover meat, fish, or fowl make a salad the centerpiece of a substantial, nutritious meal.

Fourth on my lunch list is the lengthy luncheon blowout, a sadly disappearing custom. Such lunches are among my fondest eating memories. There was the time when, after two grueling weeks producing the Montreal Comedy Festival (which I did for nine years), I came back to Brooklyn, completely beat from high-pressure show business. I called my neighbor Henry Cox, and we walked over to Gage and Tollner, a Victorian-era gaslight restaurant in downtown Brooklyn typical of East Coast seafood- and chophouses of a bygone time. The African American wait staff all wore black uniforms with gold stripes denoting their years of service (no one had been there fewer than twenty years).

We drank martinis followed by two dozen oysters, then fresh crab sautéed in butter and sherry, creamed spinach, a bottle of white Burgundy, and, for dessert, homemade gingerbread. When we requested Cognac and cigars (this was in the pre-verboten days for smoking in restaurants), the waiter beamed a fraternal smile and said, "It is a pleasure to serve two men who know how to enjoy lunch!" I only have such lunches a handful of times a year, but in an era where we are constantly at the mercy of schedules that demand we accomplish too many things in too few hours, it is empowering and enjoyable to make a command decision to shut down the day and devote a few hours to pure pleasure.

In Europe and South America, lunch is often the big meal of the day. Long and languid, perhaps followed by a siesta, it is one of the great pleasures of traveling, and usually among the first experiences recounted—even before art masterpieces. After a few weeks of following this kind of schedule abroad, the surprising thing is so many people remark that they actually lost weight on their travels. According to Lisa Sasson, a professor of nutritional studies at NYU who leads students on an annual gastro-tour of Italy, part of the explanation for this is that in the Mediterranean countries even fancy cuisine is served in smaller portions than American restaurant food. Equally important, it is uncomplicated, relying on fresh, whole ingredients rather than flavor-boosting calorie-heavy sauces: i.e., filling, not fattening. Of course, another slimming factor in tourism is that we Americans abroad tend to walk ourselves into the ground, checking off a to-do list of all the art and architecture of the Old World.

An occasional over-the-top lunch in Brooklyn or Bologna may seem like a contradiction of the tenets of CI. But Culinary Intelligence is not a moral code: it is a way to eat better most days without putting on weight. Every once in a while, a long, leisurely meal at a nice restaurant, or at home on a Sunday afternoon, feels so good that the sense of well-being it engenders is worth the extra calories. So have that shrimp cocktail, and the Dover sole or extra-thick pork chop, and a glass or two of fine Bordeaux. Wine or a cocktail has been known to help seal many deals: from business transactions to marriage proposals.

Part III: Dinnertime: The Kierkegaard Diet

For most people, the main food event of the day is dinner. While breakfast is often a hurried prelude to getting out the door, and lunch sandwiched, as it were, into a busy workday schedule, at suppertime we're off the clock. It's a chance to relax, get creative at the stove, have a cocktail, maybe some hors d'oeuvres. You feel a little looser and less pressured.

These are all good things.

What is not so good is when your culinary conscience decides it also deserves the rest of the day off. It figures that since you've been a responsible eater all day you have "earned the right" to have a double bourbon, and cheese, and a steak, and wine, and potatoes, and some pie, and, oh yeah, while you're at it, a scoop of ice cream. In terms of calories, a classic full dinner is like a car loaded with every available option: the cost, whether in money or in calories, is a budget buster.

If you let dinner just "happen," you will find yourself on a weight-gain treadmill. Without a plan, dinner can easily become another form of mindless eating. Having a plan doesn't require you to write out the week's menu in advance, like a schedule from the dietitian at your grade-school cafeteria. In my early years, those meals were so bad; it may explain my aversion to schedules. Even at age eight, I knew that Friday's regular meal at Redwood School in West Orange, New Jersey—a hamburger bun with ketchup and melted Velveeta—was straining credulity when they called it a "pizza burger." But putting aside irritating childhood food memories, it is helpful to have an overview of dinner in the context of a week's worth of dining and a conceptual grasp of what constitutes a smart plan.

In considering a strategy for dinners, figure that weekends

tend to include heftier meals than the workweek. It's also a reasonable bet that you'll have at least one weekend meal at a restaurant, which always entails a tension between the chef's wish to achieve the maximum effect—calories be damned—and your desire to eat something that tastes great, but isn't super-fattening.

The restaurant meal will probably include meat, fish, or poultry. Likewise, one of your at-home weekend meals could feature the same type of entrée. That leaves five meals to think about preparing during the rest of the week. I'm not big on take-out, in part because I enjoy cooking and in part because take-out is often heavy on sugar, salt, fat, and processed ingredients. I will make an occasional exception for a great take-out roast chicken.

Filling in the weekdays, my playbook calls for one at-home meal with meat or chicken as a featured ingredient, another with fish, usually one pasta-based meal, one whole-grain risotto, and a vegetable-and-bean ragù. For a quickie, green salad with dark bread, a couple of cheeses, and a slice or two of ham or salami. Homemade soup with a salad is yet another simple option.

A critical element in devising an enjoyable and livable plan of action is plenty of vegetables. Let the best of what is available be your guide. So, if the week's visit to the greenmarket has yielded some nice zucchini and green peas, use them as a side dish or to dress up pasta or a risotto. Pump up the FPC with sautéed shallots, garlic, hot pepper, and a bit of bacon from your larder.

This overview of a typical week breaks down as follows:

- Meat
- Poultry
- Fish
- Pasta (farro or hard durum-semolina)

- Whole-grain risotto (farro, barley, quinoa, red or black rice)
- Beans (lentils, chickpeas, white beans) made with vegetables, sausage, or bacon
- Salad
- An omelet or frittata
- Soup
- Leftovers, touched up

If you follow this schedule to the letter every week, and if you throw in a restaurant meal, it adds up to an eleven-day week. More practically, consider this list as a rough outline from which to pick and choose, a group of choices that emphasizes variety.

Though I am not in any way opposed to meat (I love it), it is a fact that meat every day—and lots of it—ends up in a calorie-rich diet. The trencherman portions of meat—make that all foods—idealized in frat-boy sports commercials (gooey oversized pizzas, cheese-and-bacon breakfast sandwiches, sweetly sauced shrimp with creamy pasta) are all too big. We have come to feel cheated with smaller—previously normal-sized—portions. We equate value with quantity. This big-plate mentality is true of every meal, but it is especially dangerous at dinner, because we take for granted that it's going to be the heaviest meal of the day. Now it has become super-extra-heavy.

Big portions are not merely a USA problem. If I had any doubts about that, Francis Mallmann, the Argentine chef with whom I wrote *Seven Fires,* cleared that up one Christmas Day.

"I'll take care of the meat," he said. "You do the rest."

In our holiday household, "the rest" is our version of the Full Monty as it appears in *The River Cottage Meat Book,* Hugh Fearnley-Whittingstall's passionate and eclectic volume: glazed carrots, braised leeks, steamed Savoy cabbage, roasted Brussels sprouts with figs and bacon, Yorkshire pudding.

Francis arrived with a *huge* rib roast in tow: sixty pounds of raw meat and bone.

"For Chrissake, Francis, who do you think is going to eat all this meat?" I asked. "Counting my parents, your wife, and my brothers' families, we are only fourteen people!"

Without irony he answered, "In Argentina we figure four pounds per person."

Although the average North American's meat consumption doesn't measure up to Argentine gaucho standards, we eat a lot of it, and we have come to expect to have a lot of it on the plate when we treat ourselves to a restaurant meal. Or, more precisely, we expect a lot of everything, and the restaurants oblige.

At home, it's easier to control portion size: don't load up the plate, and don't bring the whole platter of meat to the table. If all you have to do is reach out and spear another slice of lamb, or another chicken leg, you are likely to do so. On the other hand, if you bring all the vegetables you have prepared to the table, you are equally likely to satisfy yourself with filling vegetables, but not at great caloric expense. If you still feel the need to eat more, have a green salad after the main course, rather than before. "Salads, not seconds" is a good rule at home. In a restaurant, a salad is a good preemptive move in place of rich appetizers.

The big-portion mind-set has very noticeably been applied to pasta, which used to be a modest starter course. As a result of the fat-phobic carb craze of the last few decades, it has grown into a big meal. The pasta that most people consume is made from processed white flour. Cheese-heavy sauces add hundreds of fat calories. In truth, no one needs to "carb up" on pasta by eating a half-pound serving. Anyone who does that with regularity can't expect to take weight off and keep it off.

Mario Batali, who is a universally acknowledged pasta expert, told me, "I think the key to understanding how you can really enjoy pasta is to eat sixty grams, about two ounces. It's a nice portion, and that's how Italians eat it. They don't sit down and have a pound of pasta for three people. They have six or seven forkfuls, and that's the first course, and it's usually not with meat, it's usually with vegetables or oil, maybe some shellfish, maybe even a little pancetta. And then the rest of the meal is a small portion of protein and a nice bunch of vegetables. It's much better to eat three small plates of something than one big plate of just one thing. You get ultimate satisfaction when you eat that way."

Good advice, but it should be taken with a dose of realism. No American eats two ounces of pasta. I make a half-pound for two people and hope to save at least a lunch's worth of leftovers. In terms of volume, the food probably takes up as much room on my plate as it did when I ate more pasta per serving, but now that volume includes more caramelized vegetables, some crisped prosciutto, sautéed pepper, squash, wilted greens, chickpeas. I follow the same formula for risottos and for dishes based on lentils or beans. They need the extra flavor of onions, peppers, spices, bacon. Without these, grains and beans are boring, and, without more FPC, no one is going to keep them in a diet plan.

Serving smaller portions doesn't mean you should cook less food. Actually, it makes sense to cook more than one meal's worth of many recipes, because, as I've already mentioned, you can do so much with the leftovers. Look at it this way: Lentils cooked in red wine with caramelized vegetables will take about forty-five minutes of chopping, sautéing, and simmering whether you make one batch or two. The next day, take one link of Italian sausage, cook it, roughly dice it, and mix with the warmed-over lentil stew, and you are guaranteed a meal at least as rich as, and probably more deeply flavored than, it was in yesterday's incarnation.

Likewise, if you go to the trouble of roasting chicken, it takes only a little more work to roast two. Next day you'll have great chicken to add to a salad, or to slice and place atop a piece of toasted dark bread along with some mashed avocado, crunchy sea salt, and lime juice. It is no less pleasing, and with far fewer calories, than a deli sandwich or wrap.

The CI approach to the evening repast requires letting go of our prevailing conception of dinner—a substantial meal, usually the largest of the day. Think instead of what, in the nineteenth century, was called "supper": a light, savory meal. Except for the occasional dinner party, there's no need for a multicourse slalom that begins with cocktails and hors d'oeuvres (often very high in fat and calories), climaxing in a big hunk of flesh alongside potatoes and a vegetable, then winding down with a rich dessert.

Cocktails are dessert-in-a-glass: save them for special occasions. But a couple of glasses of wine or beer taken with the meal can make the experience of eating more pleasurable. Just as with pasta, the goal is to limit your intake rather than eliminate it. You will have no fun if you keep checking your internal calorie meter with every gulp. You'll do much better if you set a limit: two glasses of wine or beer. In fact, when beer is served with food rather than by itself, I find just one bottle is usually all I need.

Although the Danish philosopher Søren Kierkegaard did not have diet in mind when he wrote, "Purity of heart is to will one thing," it nonetheless suggests an intelligent and simple approach when applied to dinner: eat just one main course (including vegetables), followed by a green salad. I may still feel the urge for dessert, but a piece of fruit and two bites of chocolate usually does it for me. Most important, I'll get up from the table satisfied but not stuffed, and please remember, even if the evening meal is the last one of the day, it's not your Last Supper.

Snacks

Fruit kept me going for 140 years once. I was on a very strict diet. Mainly nectarines. I love that fruit. Half a peach, half a plum: it's a helluva fruit.

—*Mel Brooks,* The 2000 Year Old Man

Tell me how a person snacks and I can tell a lot about their Culinary Intelligence. Before you reach for that donut/scone/granola bar/Terra chip, bear in mind that humans did not evolve to eat constantly, like grazing cattle. We adapted to nutritionally dense food. We store fat very efficiently. Snacks weren't an issue in bygone days, when families (usually Mom) prepared their own food. There simply wasn't enough time to throw together three meals along with another three or four quick munchies to quiet midmorning, midafternoon, mid-study-hall, mid-commute hunger pangs. But with more and more women in the workforce, and more convenience foods offered outside the home at every turn, we are a nation that eats all through the day—whether we need to or not, whether we are hungry or not. We have become conditioned to eat everywhere at any time.

In meeting the opportunities presented by nonstop eating, modern commerce seeks to satisfy us with the coffee break, pizza by the slice, "emergency" candy bars kept in a desk drawer, small bags of trail mix that—for some reason, though surely not a nutritional one—are said to be four or five servings, but which are usually consumed by one person at one time, to the tune of six or seven hundred calories.

Even if you are mindful about portion size and eliminating processed food at meals, you can easily consume a whole day's worth of calories in snacks. Consider the following snack options:

24 almonds = 170 calories
1 apple = 80 calories
1 Starbucks Organic Vegan Fruit Scone = 310 calories
1-ounce bag Original Terra Chips = 140 calories
1 peach = 60 calories
Half 450-ml bottle Odwalla Mango Tango = 150 calories
1 banana = 120 calories

The whole foods on this list—almonds, peaches, bananas, apples—are better choices, and usually cheaper. Even though the processed snacks have healthy-sounding names, they are developed in laboratories and made in factories, which is a sufficient reason for me to take a pass.

The fact remains that you snack, I snack, we all snack. The danger, for a stay-at-home writer, is that every time I walk by the fridge I could easily open it and scan the contents—more out of the need for something to do than from any real hunger. Likewise, it's very easy, without thinking, to grab a handful of the almonds or pecans that Melinda keeps on hand for baking or adding to cereal.

At home, at least you have a say in what your choices are. On the job, you're at the mercy of the rulers of Fast Food Nation. Every convenience store is crammed with processed high-calorie foods. For example, consider the mini-mart in central Pennsylvania that my younger daughter, Lily, and I pulled into on our way home from a fishing trip. It was the sweet spot in the year, July, when summer's fruits and vegetables have come into season, but you wouldn't have guessed that from the shelves in the little market. The only thing local was the newspaper. I roamed the aisles searching for something nonprocessed without heaps of fat or sugar. Cumulatively, I've spent a few months of my life walking up and down similar aisles at airports, at rest stops on the New York Thruway, at newspaper stands in Manhattan, and gas stations from coast to coast. It's always the same sad story: too many sweet, fat, and salty calories.

After a typically dispiriting survey, I chose an eight-ounce bag of almonds, knowing, on the one hand, that nobody *needs* to eat an entire eight ounces of almonds (almost thirteen hundred calories). But a couple of handfuls have a lot of protein, and not-terrible-for-you fat. Throw in an apple and some water and you're set for a few hours.

"Congratulations, you picked the only healthy thing in the store," the friendly lady at the cash register said with a co-conspirator's smile.

She was probably right. If I had wanted to survive on a diet of potato chips, I had come to the right place: in addition to plain old salted chips, I could have chosen barbecue-flavored, which I've always found to be a puzzler. How do you barbecue a potato chip? The answer, I guess, was to be found on the label, which listed a number of chemical tongue-twisters, including "imitation woodsmoke." How can that not be a little carcinogenic? Or, if you're not in the mood for barbecue flavor, what about green-onion-and-sour-cream chips (notable for the absence of both onion and sour cream)? Or nacho-flavored chips, which, for some reason that has nothing to do with an actual nacho, have an aroma that you pick up downwind of a metal smelter? Seen in this light, the favorite snack food of Tina Fey's character on

30 Rock doesn't seem so far-fetched: *sabor de soledad*—the taste of loneliness—made with real *essencia del toro* (bull semen)!

To tempt my sweet tooth, the mini-mart displayed dozens of different candies whose main ingredient was refined cane sugar or high-fructose corn syrup, often both. Among them, a cornucopia of chocolate candy bars, none of which listed real chocolate—the pulverized seeds of the cacao fruit—as their principal ingredient. Cold beverages were almost all soft drinks, sports drinks, diet soda, milk, and beer. I reached for what I took to be a bottle of water and was grateful when my cashier friend pointed out that what I thought was pure water was in fact enhanced with "fruit flavorings": unsurprisingly, there was no specific fruit enumerated in the cheery cursive label that looked like a sign on a kindergarten bulletin board. Finally, tucked in a corner of the bottom shelf of the cooler, I encountered a few bottles of plain pure water.

I've acted out this same script hundreds of times, hoping to discover a plot twist that results in a few more good choices, but it's always the same. In every mini-mart I have ever visited, the most unprocessed and least chemically laden foods are usually nuts (or trail mixes that include nuts and dried fruits, but don't kid yourself that the ones with M&M's are health food). If you can find it, plain yogurt sprinkled with some nuts and dried fruits is a good light meal, or at least it can tide you over until your next real meal. If there is only fruit-flavored yogurt, I eat the unflavored part on top, or only stir in a little bit of the sugary fruit from the bottom of the container.

This brings me to the category of health/energy bars, which take up an increasing amount of shelf space wherever snacks are sold. I am of two minds about them. The better ones contain many of the same ingredients as good breakfast cereals, but almost all health bars are sweeter.

Once you recognize this, it's a short jump to the realization that a health bar is actually an aspirational cookie: delivering the fun of a cookie, while reaping all the good-behavior points of eating a health food. Though the best of these products are made from whole natural ingredients, they rely on fat, salt, and sugar to varying degrees, and the combination does nothing to combat our tendency to satisfy cravings with this trinity of first resort.

When I don't have time for a meal in the morning, or when I am about to board an airplane, where the food choices are worse, or when I am driving on a road where all the food stops are twenty miles apart and every one of them is a fast-food franchise, one of these bars is an okay option. There's no reason to eat them regularly between meals at home as a way to satisfy a cookie craving. Yet that is what I often found myself doing: I would have one as a pick-me-up at midmorning or midafternoon. At such times, I would start by making a shot of espresso, either because I needed a jolt or simply because it was something to do by way of taking a break. Bitter espresso calls for a sweet balance. A Kashi bar provides it, but I probably would be better off sweetening my coffee with a half spoonful of sugar, with 130 fewer calories.

So where does this leave me when hunger strikes and it is not yet mealtime? Apples, even when not in season locally, fill me up, and have pleasing crunch and nuanced sweetness. Though it is hard to beat a New York State Macoun in September, in midwinter and early spring trucked-in Fujis, Galas, Granny Smiths, and Honey Crisps are quite good. Likewise, clementines, blood oranges, and grapefruit, even though shipped in the winter from Florida, Texas, or California, are nutritious whole foods. From May through September, I'm big on local berries and fruits such as peaches, nectarines, plums, or melons from local farms. These whole foods will hold me for a couple of hours of writing, or through a workout at the gym, which is all you can ask of any snack.

Sometimes, when you have eaten mindfully all day, your food superego will kick in with a rationalization for consuming a few hundred unnecessary calories.

"Gee whiz," you tell yourself, "don't I deserve a couple of scoops of butter pecan? I behaved myself—give me a break!"

Strike that thought. "Behaved" is a judgmental word, better suited to describing the dynamic between child and parent than that between an adult and superego. Bad behavior, in the infantile scenario, brings punishment. Good behavior earns reward. This is a boneheaded basis for a grown-up's diet. Guilt is not an eating plan.

You don't have to choose between nutrition and pleasure, but you do have to choose between bad nutrition and pleasure. I took off a lot of weight and kept it off, but I still derive great pleasure from food.

It is never simply a matter of saying, "Listen to your body," although that sounds reassuring in a New Age kind of way. Your body got you into this mess in the first place. It likes the combination of sugar and salt and fat. It has a million generations of ancestors in its Darwinian cheering section screaming, "Go for it!"

What we have at work here is the Offset Fallacy: the idea that if you eat a healthful diet and you exercise, this somehow puts calories in the bank and earns the right to consume food that is high in salt, fat, and sugar.

I employed a form of the Offset Fallacy long before my diet issues surfaced. When I was excused (fired) from *National Lampoon* in my early thirties, rather than return to the cab-driving profession, I spent about a hundred days a year clambering over boulders, fishing my way up swift-running streams, bird-shooting in the crisp, colorful afternoons of Catskill autumns, cross-country skiing in the Adirondacks, canoeing on hot summer days. I earned a modest living writing about these adventures. I looked upon my new vocation as creating escapist literature for people with real jobs. My preferred outdoorsman's breakfast was coffee (in hot weather, a Coca-Cola), a Marlboro, and a Snickers bar. "What the hell?" I told myself. "You burn a lot of calories running up and down mountainsides shooting at grouse, woodcock, and the occasional rabbit."

This line of reasoning proved to be a potent stimulus for the Offset Fallacy. Bookending the day that my sportsman's breakfast began, I had the perfect answer to the hunger and thirst that the day's physical activity built up. First, a very cold can of Budweiser for the thirst. Then, for the hunger, a bag of Nacho Cheese Doritos.

Let's consider the flawed nutritional reasoning that led me to this snack. I had long ago taken it as an article of faith that a mile of jogging and, by extension, an activity such as bushwhacking through berry tangles and abandoned orchards, shotgun in hand, compensated for a can of beer. This stratagem had been promulgated by Lee Eisenberg, a friend who was the editor of *Esquire* magazine, which I felt granted him sufficient authority to dispense dietary advice. Lee's actual formula was: one mile equals one beer.

By my calculation, I met Lee's caloric benchmark when I traversed two or three miles of hillside, running after a Labrador retriever that was locked onto the scent of a game bird. As for the Doritos, they went along with the beer, and I reasoned that they abound in salt, and I had lost much of that through perspiration; plus, they are made from corn, which is a nice vegetable, and cheese, which has healthy protein. Clearly, and I was clueless, and as any of you who are fans of Nacho Cheese Doritos know, once I started to eat them, I was destined to finish the whole bag. Thus, without giving it much—or any—thought, I consumed at least seven hundred calories: for a snack, not even a meal.

Pretty soon I no longer needed the mountain walk; completing any outdoor activity proved to be a sufficient stimulus. The Offset Fallacy had morphed into the Bud and Doritos Reflex.

Eating without thinking is often that way: you keep putting food in your mouth. Sitting in front of the television eating popcorn, potato chips, Raisinets, or cheese-bomb pizzas is a monumental waste of calories. Movie-theater snacks are no better. The sodas are bigger than anything you would pour for yourself, popcorn comes in buckets, and the candy is sold in packages that are, likewise, larger than anything you would normally choose.

Put aside the question whether or not any of these foods are nutritious, which for the most part they are not. The real question is, do you really need that much food in order to enjoy a show? Do you need any? Even if you do need some food, made-for-TV (or movie) snacks are the junkiest of junk foods. At best, they satisfy a craving for a brief moment. They are high in calories, and they are hyper-palatable, so that any normal human being who starts by eating one chip, one peanut, one Hershey's kiss, will keep eating . . . and eating . . . and eating.

You can exercise at the gym four days a week. You can pass up French fries, eat whole-grain bread, organically raised chickens that are fed wild blueberries, and quinoa that is harvested after being blessed by an Inca priest, but every time you sit down in front of the TV with a bowl of chips, or settle into a seat at the movies with a box of Sour Patch Kids (I love them), you wreak havoc with your caloric balance sheet.

Don't go there.

CHAPTER VII When You're Away from Home

Any American who has driven a car more than fifty miles and tried to find something to pacify a hunger pang can tell the same story: it's hard, and sometimes damn near impossible, to eat a healthy diet on the road. You can't help being tempted to give in and have a Big Mac. Or, if you don't surrender, you drive some more until you are so stomach-growlingly hungry that you capitulate and wolf down two Big Macs. And while you're at it, some fries too. And—what the heck?—you might as well wash it down with a soda.

It doesn't matter what part of the country you are in; as a people, we may be divided by politics, or the kinds of music we like, but we are united in the sameness and the prevailing unhealthfulness of the food options we are presented with when we stray far from home.

The situation has not improved very much since the early part of the twentieth century, when Christine Fredericks mourned the loss of gastronomic diversity in America:

> I have eaten in Florence, Alabama, in Logan, Utah, in Mansfield, Ohio and Penobscot, Maine. Is there any difference in the meals served in one locality or another? No. The customer will always sit down to the same old steak, or canned beans, bottle catsup, French fries or Adam and Eve on a raft [old-time restaurant slang for two poached eggs on toast]. Where, I ask you, is the sweet potato pone of Maryland for a slice of which General Lee would walk a mile? Where is the genuine clam chowder of New England? Gone, or rapidly disappearing under an absolutely false effort of the restaurateur to standardize his food.

Today, that lament is even more to the point. To illustrate this, I could pick any road trip I have taken in the last twenty years and, with subtle differences—maybe more fried stuff in the South, more chili with spaghetti in the Midwest (known to natives as a chili mac)—it's pretty much the same story. Take, for example, a road trip that Melinda and I made across Wyoming and the Great Plains en route to a Fourth of July family reunion in Rockford, Illinois.

The mountains still wore their spring mantle of white. The bottom lands were green as the Forest of Arden. Wildflowers carpeted the landscape for a thousand miles.

We started on an optimistic note, stocking our cooler with good inexpensive wine from Osco Drug, in Bozeman, Montana. Maybe this isn't a surprising wine venue to you, if you are from one of the towns in our nation's heartland that has an Osco, but I had never thought to go wine shopping in an establishment that also has aisles full of laxatives, antacids, mouthwashes, eyebrow pencils, and condoms.

Our first day's drive—through Yellowstone Park, then on to Cody, Wyoming, and east—was breathtaking in its beauty, but it did not offer much in the way of food: we subsisted on trail mix and fresh fruit. That evening I ate a bar burger, bun removed, and a martini (with two olives as the vegetable course). Next day our tourism goal was sunset at Devils Tower. You may recall it as the monolith that attracted Richard Dreyfuss's character to a rendezvous with the aliens in *Close Encounters of the Third Kind.*

The real-life Devils Tower is, indeed, spectacular: the truncated cone of a volcano that never punched its way through the earth's crust, it looms in the distance for an hour before you arrive at its base. The approach precludes conversation beyond awestruck whispers, as if you were in the presence of a great work of art in a church. The looping road offers views of the stillborn volcano in an increasingly massive aspect, until, finally, the blue haze that surrounds faraway things disappears and the fluted sides of the rock formation come into sharp focus. For a moment you can't help but think that this looming tower anchors the sky to the earth.

Though it was the beginning of the summer tourist season, there wasn't much of a crowd. We strolled around the base, taking a few steps, halting, staring upward, and marveling. In the afternoon updrafts, hawks and vultures wheeled silently a thousand feet overhead. Two climbers, about three-quarters of the way up the Tower, were just specks on the mass of basalt. You could hear the *ping ping* of their hammers as they inched their way up.

We had been told to be sure to stay for the last moments of

alpenglow, so we found a bench with a good view of the Tower's southwestern face. A middle-aged couple sat down beside us.

"Where are you from?" Melinda asked.

"Kansas," they answered. The man added wistfully, "We wanted to see this one more time before we're gone."

Kind of a downer sentiment for such an inspiring sight, especially from a guy who didn't look much older than I was. I turned back to watch the rock light up and glow in the sun's last flame-pink rays. Then, like a scene fading out in a movie, the color drained from the tableau, and starry night fell. We walked back to the car and thought about dinner. We'd passed a number of roadside places on the way in. For sure we'd find something.

You'd think that at 9 p.m. in Wyoming, where Devils Tower is the icon on the state's license plate, there would have been places nearby where one could eat.

There were, but the options did not extend beyond a few raucous roadhouses, their parking lots crammed with tricked-out Harley-Davidsons.

This should not have surprised us. Everywhere we went that week, within a two-hundred-mile radius, there were men in black leather chaps and studded leather vests, bandannas tied around their heads (often to hide a balding pate), and girlfriends or wives similarly leathered. The occasion was the annual Harley hajj to Sturgis, South Dakota.

Melinda agreed that a bar full of bikers and the prospect of head-banging heavy-metal did not feel like the right spiritual segue from our transcendental sunset mood.

Thinking back to being on the road in Europe, Melinda suggested, "Let's pick up some bread and cold cuts and cheese at the store, and open a bottle of our nice wine." This is a good plan of action in Europe—a loaf of good bread, some fresh fruit, a bit of ham or sausage—but in the little town where we overnighted just outside the Black Hills of South Dakota we found far fewer wine/cheese/cold cuts options than in Siena or Toulouse, which is why our only recourse was the mini-mart. Back in our room at the Days Inn motel, we ate "dinner": a terrific Provençal rosé along with pickles, Triscuits, Cracker Barrel cheese, and a chocolate bar (Hershey's Dark with almonds). It was the best we could do.

The next evening after we toured the Black Hills, marveling at the primeval scenery and its herds of bison and pronghorn antelope, we made a reservation at a highly recommended restaurant. Nice place, nice people, but strange combinations of ingredients. Tenderloin of beef, buffalo, and wapiti (that's elk, for those who don't speak the Cree language) with "Peanut Sweet Soy Relish" left me wondering, "Why a Peanut Sweet Soy Relish?" Surely the Cree would never have tried such a bizarre combination. In fact, why use sweet-soy anything when you are trying to show off three different meats? Could it be that we have become so accustomed to franchises' serving sweet glazes as compensation for tasteless farm-raised shrimp, or equally dull factory-farm pork, that we have come to expect it on all of our meats, even superior ones that don't need the help?

Isn't the point of a good restaurant that it should serve ingredients so deeply flavored that they don't need to be overpowered with condiment fixes? Or how about medallions of Black Angus with blue-cheese demi-glace? Again, why hide a premium ingredient under a super-strong cheese sauce guaranteed to obliterate any subtlety in the flavor of the beef?

I do not in any way mean to single out this one restaurant. The meat was good, the staff too. You run into the same well-intentioned attempts at gourmet food everywhere. In Alaska I was once invited by some chef friends from the lower forty-eight to help them judge a seafood cook-off. The previous day, we all had gone fishing and caught about a ton (well, actually closer to four hundred pounds) of salmon and halibut. That night, I mise-en-placed ingredients as directed while the chefs—John Besh, Robert Wiedmaier, and Randy Lewis—prepared our fish, along with freshly gathered chanterelles, wild dandelion greens, and raspberries.

At the cook-off, instead of utilizing the local bounty, many of the competing chefs tarted up their entries with harissa, jicama salsa, mangoes. I don't know if it's because of the influence of shows like *Iron Chef* and *Top Chef,* but for some years there has been a move afoot toward ambitious, fussy presentations, exotic ingredients, and weird combinations that far outrun the capabilities of many chefs. If picking a winner hadn't been required, we might not have chosen one. Unless there is a compelling reason to do otherwise, when combining ingredients in the kitchen (or ordering items off a menu) you'd do well to remember the mantra that Tom Colicchio shared with me many years ago, when I was writing about the opening of Gramercy Tavern: "If it grows together, it goes together." Not that there aren't creative combinations out there waiting to be tried, but, for example, cooking oranges with potatoes is probably not one of them.

Even if all the ambitious food you encounter is oversauced and overcomplicated, and franchise food is loaded with, for want of a better term, "bad stuff," you still have options for a decent road meal. On longer trips, when you are out on the open road and there is a village or small town just off the highway, you stand a good chance of finding a reasonably okay nonfranchise place. If there is still a Main Street in town, look for the café with two or three pickup trucks parked in front and—an even better sign—a table full of retirees, often viewable through the window, gabbing away.

At most, this reconnaissance effort might cost you a half-hour in detour time. I guarantee you'll find that America still has plenty of nice coffee shops, diners, and small restaurants. There's often a soup of the day, or steak and eggs, or my go-to sandwich, a whole-wheat BLT with a scrambled egg on top, which gives you vegetables, whole-grain bread, and an egg. During our trip, we came upon a sweet little café in an old Nebraska town with a gabled and turreted redbrick courthouse from the days when the railroads still came through and ranching was the source of many local fortunes. In the middle of Nebraska, on a hot afternoon, a BLT on a shady street always beats a food court in a mall hands-down. The local bacon was super.

In Thornton, Iowa, the last meal on our road trip was also the best. We had been invited to a cookout out at the farm of my friend Paul Willis, the sustainably minded former Peace Corps volunteer who became a pig farmer and founder of the Niman Ranch Pork Company. We arrived about an hour before sundown on July 3. A few families had assembled around a campfire on a little hill overlooking a patch of prairie that Paul and his wife, Phyllis, have restored to its natural state of wild grasses, flowers, and "prairie potholes"—rain-fed ponds that attract migrating waterfowl in spring and autumn.

The prairie was covered with wildflowers: bluestem and Indian grass, shooting stars and blazing stars, heartbeats, Golden Alexander, pale-purple cornflower, death camas, butterfly milkweed, and rattlesnake master.

"Rattlesnake master?" I asked.

"Yes. There's two stories about it. Either it attracts rattlesnakes or it keeps them away. I've never seen a rattlesnake on my farm, so it must keep them away."

He waited two or three beats, and then, with a deadpan delivery worthy of Bob Newhart, added, "Of course, there really aren't rattlesnakes here anyway."

The cookout/potluck dinner featured a salad of greens picked that afternoon. I believe there was macaroni salad as well. Definitely some potato salad. No Iowa corn on the cob, though, because, as the saying goes in the Midwest, corn is only "knee-high by July." The main event was pork burgers made from a recipe handed down by Phyllis's Danish grandmother. The fragrant, scrumptious meat was free-range pork raised on the Willis farm: *molto* porky with great depth of flavor.

But I had eaten pork from the Willis farm in the past, so it was welcome but not unexpected. The surprise palate-popper was a plate of boiled radishes. To me those two words—"boiled radishes"—sound like something a Woody Allen character might have said to get a laugh as he disparaged American (i.e., non–New York) food. But those boiled radishes, moments from the garden, sliced in two, seasoned with kosher salt, and drizzled with olive oil, are still among our favorite food memories from the whole trip. Fresh, simple, whole ingredients.

Lightning bugs flickered on and off in the gathering dusk. The kids added to Mother Nature's light show, waving sparklers in the air and giggling at silly jokes. They roasted marshmallows by the campfire: not exactly whole, unprocessed ingredients, but, after all, they were kids and it was almost the Fourth of July . . . almost. A fitting American end to a journey from the Rockies to the Mississippi.

If there is one dependable salvation to eating on the road, it is ethnic food. Traditional recipes, especially among recent immigrants, haven't had time to be deconstructed, then chemically reconstructed, and industrially processed into the mainstream of American food. For this reason, I look for ethnic whenever I am traveling. I remember, a few years back, stopping to make a business call while driving through North Carolina en route to a gathering of former tobacco farmers whom Paul Willis had enlisted in a sustainable hog-rearing program.

I pulled off the highway. It was early November on a clear fall day. The fields and orchards had already been harvested, but there was still plenty to be gleaned by the convoys of ducks and geese making their way south.

A lone country store sat next to a shaded parking lot where I dialed in to a conference call. I paced up and down, paying little attention to my surroundings. But my nose remained on duty. In much the same way that you hear your name being called in a dream and then wake to find that someone is in fact calling you, I awoke and responded to the meaty aroma of roast pork and an onion-laden fresh-herb smell.

I walked up to the front door of a wooden building that looked as if it had once been a farmhouse. The clapboard on the first story was painted white; the second floor, which I guessed to be the living quarters, was a deep green, the same color as the stand of graceful pines that marked the property line around the building. An RC Cola sign hung in the window, round as a bottle top, pitted with age: the real thing, definitely not designer-inspired kitsch intended to give an old-timey feel to a theme restaurant that you'd find beside a heavily trafficked exit ramp.

A hand-lettered menu board, in a haphazard mix of upper- and lowercase script, solved the mystery of the come-hither aroma. "*Comida mexicana,*" it promised, and beneath that headline "*tacos, tamales, carne asada, pollo, coloraditos.*" A short lady with a long ponytail and a singsong Spanish accent took my order: one *carne asada* taco (strips of grilled skirt steak) and another of *coloraditos* (chunks of seasoned pork). She warmed two corn tortillas on the grill, and, cupping them in her hand, filled one with beef and the other with pork, topping both with homemade *pico de gallo* (diced fresh tomato, onion, parsley, cilantro, jalapeño, and garlic). In case I liked it spicier, she pointed to a bowl of green-tomato-and-jalapeño salsa.

It's the same all over America. In farm communities and in cities and towns, the growing Latino population, eager for the familiar tastes of home, have given rise to small restaurants, roadside food trucks, and grocery stores with food made according to time-honored recipes—from scratch—with ingredients that are recognizable as food, rather than puzzling chemicals.

Latino food is the most prevalent ethnic option one encounters in traveling the United States, but it is by no means the only one. For example, if you ever tire of the food in New Orleans—and a steady diet of even the most wonderful po'boys, beignets, and jambalaya can leave you longing for a change of pace—there is a large community of Vietnamese immigrants and their first-generation offspring who earn their livelihood as Gulf Coast fishermen. Independent Vietnamese American restaurants and stores often sell freshly made recipes based on the shrimp, fish, squid, pork, vegetables, and condiments that make Southeast Asian cuisine so light and so appealing. A thousand miles upstream, at the other end of the Mississippi, Minneapolis and its environs have also received a Vietnamese influx, and I am no longer surprised to find good Vietnamese food on the home turf of Rocky and Bullwinkle.

If you live in or are traveling through a region with Pakistani, Bengali, or Arab immigrants, you have your pick of still more whole-ingredient-based cuisines that have perfected the most sublime combinations of aromatic spices. They work wonders with lamb, chickpeas, fava beans, fish, okra, and other satisfying foods that you will never have the pleasure of tasting if you confine your on-the-go dining to franchises and food courts.

Rule of thumb: if you see a place with a foreign-language menu, check it out. If no one in there looks like you, *definitely* check it out even more. Don't be afraid of standing out or being different. In nearly forty years of driving in America and stopping for a bite, I have never, not once, felt unwelcome in an ethnic restaurant. In fact, quite to the contrary, I usually find that the staff and the owners are appreciative of the chance to extend their client base, and, along with their customers, they are pleased to show off their heritage.

CHAPTER VIII A Practical Guide to Restaurant Dining

Restaurants, on the road or in your hometown, present their own set of problems. Though there is definitely a nationwide trend to farm-to-table, sustainable food, the restaurateur's primary interest remains, as it has always been, to impress your palate; one surefire way is to amp up the sweet, salt, and fat components of the menu. It's not hard to consume two thousand calories at a restaurant meal, sometimes even more.

Once you settle into the comforting ambience of a restaurant, full of the aromas of delicious food, your CI defenses are down. The bonhomie of people at their leisure enjoying the company of their dining companions and their meals is infectious. "What the heck?" you tell yourself. "Might as well join in the fun."

That line of reasoning—my occupational hazard as a food writer—gained me more than thirty pounds.

When you go to a restaurant, order strategically. First have some water. In New York City, tap water piped in from the Catskills is hard to beat. You will doubtless be asked if you want to order a cocktail right away. I usually don't, although from time to time, just because I am in the mood, I might order a martini or a bourbon old-fashioned. In that event, if it's one of those restaurants that pour mixed drinks in a glass big enough to bathe a small pet, I'll ask for half a martini, even if I have to pay for the whole thing. My precise formulation is "I'd like a baby martini. You can charge me for a whole one if you want to." Sometimes they don't.

More often I'll wait for the food before I start to drink alcohol, although at a special occasion a glass of sparkling wine at the outset makes everyone feel a little more festive.

Now for the wine decision. This has both caloric and financial aspects. First the money factor: I *never* order really expensive wine. In a serious restaurant, the house white and the house red—in a bottle or a carafe—should be good and affordable. Even without the choice of a house wine, there should be some good-value bottles on the list.

Although the calories in wine are not negligible, to my way of thinking wine is a necessity. The question then becomes one of quantity and pace. If it's just two of us, half-bottles, wine by the glass, or small carafes/quartinos (quarter-liters) will get us through a meal. Be mindful that a waiter will top off your wine more often than you might. And then, when he says, "Another bottle, or would you like to move on to something different?," you are disposed to follow his suggestion. In manuals for salesmanship this is known as the Presumptive Close. Pour your own.

If we don't finish a bottle, there is no shame in taking it home. You would probably be right in assuming that the staff will drink it or cook with it if you don't. Be aware of open-container laws, though. Stick the bottle in the trunk of the car, first making sure it is well corked.

Some food goes best with beer. Chinese food is beer-friendly. Indian too. For that matter, German and Austrian also belong on the good-with-beer list. Come to think of it, beer is good with most foods. The fictional detective and gourmet Nero Wolfe thought wine was unsuitable for food and always drank beer. As Jean-Georges Vongerichten once explained to me while we were working on a story that required him to dream up new cocktails, "The bitterness and the bubbles in beer completely clean off your palate, so you are ready for the next bite of anything." Because of the calories, I try to keep it to one beer. Please note, I said I try. I don't beat myself up if I have two.

Even before I order food, I take the measure of a restaurant by one simple observation: how do they serve their bread and butter? I hope they include some dark, whole-grain bread, but if not and it's a beautiful white baguette or crusty *pan pugliese,* I'll live dangerously, break off a piece, mostly crust, and butter it—fully savoring one or two mouthfuls. The way a restaurant treats butter for the table tells you a lot about the care that it takes with other ingredients, and that, in turn, gives you a window on the underlying spirit of a place. If butter comes to the table soft, I have visions of milk curdling, oysters suffocating, and fresh produce wilting in the heat of the kitchen. Equally reproachable is hard-to-spread butter served directly from a very cold refrigerator. Rather than the carelessness or indifference that soft butter conveys, hard butter proclaims, "We are very busy, so we can't waste time coddling your little dish of butter."

Now it's time to look at the menu. Be mindful of portion

size. Huge portions are so much a part of our foodscape that we no longer notice them, or at least I didn't fully comprehend this until last summer in Manhattan. We had just seen a play in the East Village. Melinda suggested that we skip the subway and walk home. It was a lovely New York night, with a cool, velvety breeze from off the harbor, perfect for an hour's stroll. We made our way through SoHo and found ourselves walking down Hester, Grand, and Mulberry streets, the heart of Little Italy. I hadn't been there in a few years. The old landmarks were all bustling: Umberto's Clam House, where the late mafioso Joey Gallo had his final dinner before being whacked; Ferrara Bakery, Angelo's, Benito's—holdovers from an era when pasta was still called spaghetti and the word "gravy" always meant red sauce. There were also a slew of new places that looked as if they could have been flown across the ocean from contemporary Florence, Milan, Rome. Very Italian, very modern.

The décor of these new places looked authentically Italian. The waiters who picked their way among the tables that crowded the sidewalks spoke Italian. The chalkboards with the special dishes of the day were written in Italian. The wines by the glass were Italian. Yet something was out of place, non-Italian. I couldn't put my finger on it, but I knew it was there, just out of memory's reach.

Finally—aha!—I knew what was different. The plates were bigger than in Italy, and full to overflowing, heaped with mounds of food. Where a single veal cutlet is served as a *milanesa* in Milan, two were the rule here. Steaming plates of pasta that would feed four people in Trentino were served as single portions here. No three-inch squares of lasagna, as in Le Marche; instead, one-pound bricks fashioned from noodles, cheese, more cheese, and tomato sauce, with some sausage slices thrown in for good measure.

The phenomenon of portion-creep, frequently put forward to explain the leap in America's caloric intake, is often attributed to franchise foods and soft drinks. But supersizing has permeated the wider food culture. We have grown so used to king-sized servings that we have come to treat them as the norm, in much the same way that big SUVs and King Cab pickup trucks with wide seats (meant to accommodate wide-beamed drivers and passengers) came to be accepted as average-sized automobiles. To the suggestion that no one is making you eat it all, the answer is, people eat more when more food is put in front of them. It is the nature of the human animal; if they serve it, you will probably eat it.

Knowing that even many of the best restaurants serve large portions, if we are dining with another couple I'll suggest that we order two, maybe three appetizers and two entrées. For larger groups, one à-la-carte entrée per two persons is a good rule of thumb. I also like to order à-la-carte vegetables. If all this ends up being too much food, don't be embarrassed, no matter how fancy the restaurant, to ask for a doggy bag. Actually, this holds especially true in a fancy restaurant. The chef is usually happier knowing that you think the food that required so much work is worth taking home and enjoying again, rather than being scraped into the garbage.

A couple of years ago, we had planned a Christmas-season meal with friends in downtown Manhattan, at Savoy, which was a pioneering farm-to-table restaurant long before that phrase came into vogue—probably before it was invented. It sat in an unassuming nineteenth-century building straight out of Currier and Ives New York. With two working fireplaces, it was one of my favorite places in the wintertime.

My brother Bob and his wife, Doris, had come east to spend a few weeks with us and their two daughters, who live in New

York. A monster blizzard interfered with their plans to leave town for a few days, so I called the owner, Peter Hoffman, and asked if we could make our original party of four into a mini-horde of nine.

"I can handle it," he said, "but you're all going to have roast suckling pig. You can order starters and desserts separately, but I can't do nine different entrées."

As it turned out, we didn't need to order anything. The chef, Ryan Tate, took the initiative and sent out oysters, grilled octopus, homemade pâtés and charcuterie. To go with the suckling pig, which he had done up as porchetta—rolled and stuffed with fennel pollen, herbs, and garlic—the vegetables were served family-style: roast turnips with balsamic vinegar and a touch of maple syrup, roast Brussels sprouts also with balsamic vinegar, creamy and nutty cranberry beans, and braised Savoy cabbage.

We didn't have a prayer of finishing that bountiful spread, so we asked that the leftovers be packed up. For supper the next day, we sliced the porchetta and crisped it in hot canola oil, pan-roasted the Brussels sprouts and turnips, then tossed in the beans and cabbage. I put the warmed vegetable mix on serving plates and topped it with the crisped porchetta: a spot-on meal for seven, and we hadn't spent another nickel.

Most of the time, I am not in the position of having a restaurant chef do all the choosing. Under normal conditions, just like any civilian, I look over the appetizers first. With CI in mind, I keep an eye out for breadings and cheese. Breadings, as in empanadas or fried calamari, mean white flour, and, quite often, frying. That's a lot of extra calories before you even get to what's inside.

Many artisanal restaurants now make their own pâtés and charcuterie. This is a good thing, but in my case not without hazard. Because I wrote a whole book about my search for the perfect pig, the chef often sends out a platter of charcuterie. A few bites—especially with some pickled vegetables—is enough to tickle my palate. I stop there. Foie gras, another diet-buster, often appears in the appetizer section. It's quite wonderful, but it should be the occasional treat rather than a normal starter.

If there are freshly shucked oysters and clams, they always get my vote.

In a departure from my practice at home, in a restaurant I often order salad to begin the meal. It's a way to get some volume in your stomach right away, which means there is less room for what follows. Sometimes we'll order a few salads as part of the appetizer round. Although salad at home means mixed greens to me, I am happy to see restaurants moving toward more variety in salad vegetables. In the world of bistros, gastropubs, and tapas, an enormous amount of chefly creativity has gone into the salad part of the menu. Tuscan kale with a freshly made Caesar salad dressing—not stinting on anchovies—is one of my new favorites. The London chef Fergus Henderson, beloved of Anthony Bourdain for his use of offal and other "nasty bits," serves roast marrow bones on toast with a salad of onions, capers, and parsley. It's spectacular.

Always ask about the dressing. The simpler the better. Fruity vinaigrettes put me on guard. You don't need blue-cheese dressing either. Again, I'm not saying it's not delicious, but a simple vinaigrette is no less delicious, with far fewer calories and much less fat.

If the soup of the day is interesting, ask if it's made with cream or butter. If it is, you can assume it's made with a lot of both. The words "butternut-squash soup" roll comfortingly off the tongues of waiters when the first frosts of autumn come. Sounds good, but ask what's in it.

Pasta specials always are seductive, especially when they throw in words like "ragù" or "guanciale," but you don't need it for a main course, especially in the king-sized portions usually served in American restaurants. A better strategy is to treat pasta as an appetizer course and share one order among a few of you (these portions will be more like the size of a pasta course in Italy).

As for entrées, if you are avoiding White Stuff, as I try to do, ask if you can substitute something for potatoes or white rice. Restaurateurs know that including a potato in a short description of any dish increases sales. It's a subconscious comfort factor. One of New York's savviest restaurateurs—who prefers to remain anonymous—once told me, "I could sell my grandmother's ass if it had the words 'mashed potatoes' next to it."

If no substitutions are allowed, simply ask that these foods be left off your plate. And if that doesn't work, just don't eat them. Sautéed greens or beans are fine substitutes. If there are à-la-carte vegetable side dishes, ask about having any of those instead. If there is no charge, that's great, but if it costs a few bucks more, so what?

One of my restaurant bugaboos is the overly creative chef who sneaks a lot of ingredients into a sauce without telling you beforehand. I have been inflicted with otherwise fine roast lamb that was burdened with blueberry sauce, an unannounced cilantro pesto on what I thought would be a straight-ahead broiled strip steak, a sweet-savory "fusion" sauce that obliterated the taste of a plateful of scallops that were said to be fresh. How would you know if they were? Such Frankenstein creations never benefit the main ingredient. They always leave me wondering, "Why?"

You are never wrong to ask, "How is it made?" If the sauce

sounds suspicious, then request that it be put on the side. If the waiter is resistant, then "I'm allergic to cilantro" or "I'm lactose-intolerant" works like a charm.

As for dessert, I love it but I don't need it. Most restaurant desserts are heavy on some combination of sugar, flour, butter, and eggs. In terms of CI they are all pretty much the same: not great choices. If turning down dessert throws a wet blanket on a social occasion, then, if, for example, we are four people we'll ask for one or two desserts "with four straws." This usually gets a smile from the waiter, or at least neutralizes the sales pitch.

Eating out is one of the favorite pastimes of modern civilization. The opportunity to gather with friends and family for a meal is always alluring. Completely escaping the chores of shopping, cooking, and cleaning up represents a gift of time in jammed schedules. Amid all the conversation, convenience, and camaraderie, it is easy to put Culinary Intelligence aside. But I have found it equally true that if you get in the CI habit it doesn't take too much effort to keep CI in mind as you order and eat.

And remember, there is no law that says you have to finish everything on your plate.

In Conclusion: 'Tis a Gift to Be Simple

A few years ago, my family attended the first New York City concert ever given by the Shakers. Four old ladies and three younger men, from the last remaining Shaker community—in Sabbathday Lake, Maine—took the stage. The Shakers are forbidden to have sex, so they have relied on proselytizing to replenish their membership. It occurred to me that their New York debut could also be their New York farewell.

Among the songs they sang that night was "A Simple Shaker Hymn," also known as "'Tis the Gift to Be Simple."

Simplicity is chief among the Shaker virtues. It is the path to spiritual fulfillment. It is also what Culinary Intelligence comes down to. I have found that the culinary advice I value most—from people whose opinions I respect—is also quite simple.

Marion Nestle, whose book *What to Eat* deconstructs the American supermarket in clear, uncompromising, and scientifically informed terms, advises:

1. Eat real food
2. Move

In other words, diet and exercise.

Michael Pollan, whose provocative and lyric food writing has inspired millions, boiled his philosophy down to "Eat food, mostly plants, not too much."

Very simple. So is Culinary Intelligence. You don't have to write cookbooks or know famous chefs to eat healthy and well.

To Marion Nestle's second point, "Move," I'll also cast an affirmative vote. But, although exercise is important, people who rely on it to "bank calories" are probably not going to lose weight or maintain a healthy one. There's no denying that exercise makes you feel better. It's good for your heart. It burns calories. But it's not a diet. I am lucky in that I live in a big city where walking at least a mile every day is the norm. I bike and also go to the YMCA three or four times a week to work out with weights, stretch, do a little cardio. It doesn't matter all that much what exercise plan you follow, as long as your heart, your back, and your muscles can handle it. Just do something.

Nor does it matter how old you are when you rethink your diet—you just need to make the change. As I mentioned earlier, my friend Kevin Stuessi was in his forties when he changed his diet and he dropped forty-five pounds. I was in my late fifties when I reformed and am holding at minus forty pounds. Retired overweight ex-Marine Ed Keller, the father of Thomas Keller, dropped forty-five pounds when he was in his late sixties. His secret? He ate daily family meals with his son and the staff at the French Laundry: nothing fancy, just whole foods, lots of fresh fruits and vegetables.

We all followed the same commonsense diet. To give it a

label, I have called it Culinary Intelligence. "Culinary common sense" might have served just as well. It rests on three pillars:

1. Don't eat processed foods.
2. Buy the best, most full-flavored ingredients you can afford.
3. Make those ingredients even better by cooking: the surest way to maximum FPC.

The second and third rules follow from number one: cut out processed foods. Humankind did quite well for millions of years without them.

You can too.

Fourteen Recipes

I have written many cookbooks, but this is not one of them. Instead, it's an approach to food and eating. Still, I thought it would be useful to include a few recipes that exemplify how a vote for CI needn't be a commitment to unexciting, less-than-satisfying food. There is no secret to it. All that is required is the best ingredients, cooked in a way that maximizes flavor and satisfaction: ripe fruit, fresh and, for the most part, local vegetables, free-range meat and poultry, and sustainably harvested fish (preferably wild).

Although a recipe can only be as good as the ingredients that go into it, an indifferent cook can ruin them. In the hands of someone who knows how to cook, and even enjoys it, good can become better, taste richer, flavor more satisfying.

Knowing how to caramelize and brown ingredients is a quick route to delectable recipes. Extracting liquids and reducing them to concentrate flavor is another—whether it is juice drawn from the meaty interior of a steak and deposited on its crunchy crust, or water evaporating from a tomato roasted in the oven.

Developing intrinsic flavor and bringing out the taste of umami whenever possible will make for more satisfying meals without adding calories.

Braising—the art of slow cooking in stocks and wine—will pull out and marry the flavors in meat, poultry, fish, and vegetables to produce meals that will be better the second day than they are on the first. A little maturing never hurts, whether one is speaking of wine or veal stew (or your children).

It is said—though I have never fully agreed—that you can have too much of a good thing. Making two chickens instead of one, a winter's worth of oven-roasted tomatoes, or a three-night supply of braised veal shanks takes just a bit more work than making enough for one meal, but the amount of labor needed per meal plummets, taking with it the argument that we are too busy to cook very often.

Laurie Colwin wrote, in her lovely memoir *Home Cooking,* "Most things are frills—few are essential. It is perfectly possible to cook well with very little. Most of the world cooks over fire without any gadgets at all."

There is great truth in this. A good skillet, two good knives (a big one and a little one), a wooden spoon, and a few pots can turn out thousands of wonderful recipes. The truth of her words extends beyond equipment, however, to the world of technique: you don't need a culinary education and ten years on the line at Noma to make any of the following recipes—or most of my favorite recipes, for that matter. When I wrote *The Elements of Taste* with Gray Kunz, there was not one recipe in the book that required more than knowing how to chop, stir, and heat. The flavors were complicated, but the skills required were not.

Some of the following recipes are adapted from chef friends, some from other writers, some from "civilians." As is true of almost every recipe ever made, they are all the result of one cook's adding a twist to the work of cooks who have gone before. To paraphrase Isaac Newton, "If I have added something to a dish, it is because I have stood on the cookbooks of giants."

And never forget the invaluable power of serendipity. Often a recipe is the result of "making do" with the ingredients on hand. Many magnificent meals were born of laziness: "I don't feel like dragging my butt to the supermarket again, so let me see what I can dream up."

Culinary Intelligence plus Imagination: it's a simple formula, but one that can create a lifetime's worth of healthful, delicious, interesting, and nutritious meals.

Oven-Roasted Tomatoes Apart from onions, tomatoes are the most important plant for the way I cook and eat. The balance of sweet and acid is like a fruity and crisp wine. To that, add the baconlike smoky umami flavor found in true vine-ripened tomatoes, the lovely texture that they bring to a sauce or stew as they blend in with herbs and infuse meats, the caramelized crust that develops when they are roasted or sautéed at high heat. Perfection!

Some years ago, Tom Colicchio took me to his favorite sandwich shop—Melampo, in Little Italy. The proprietor was a real piece of work. People would line up at the counter and marvel at the sandwich-building skills of curmudgeonly Alessandro Gualandi. If some imported goodies on the shelves caught your eye, which they were bound to do because there were all manner of Italian delicacies, you dared not step out of line. If you did, Gualandi would bark at you, threatening that you would forfeit your place.

He assembled sandwiches with the precision of a watchmaker adjusting a fine Swiss mechanism. It was foolhardy to request substitutions or changes to any of his sandwiches. "I would not request that" was how his response came out in English, although the words he muttered under his breath sounded like the Sicilian cuss words that the Italian kids in my junior high used when angered.

It was a fine September afternoon, so Tom and I sat on a bench at the neighboring playground as we ate and chatted. On that day of notable sandwiches—mine had silky thin-sliced mortadella with roasted sweet pepper and a slice of ripe beefsteak tomato—the conversation turned to Tom's oven-roasted tomatoes. I jotted down the recipe and showed it to Melinda.

Since that day, Melinda has made roast tomatoes every weekend from mid-August through early October. We freeze them in pint or quart containers, and all through the winter we eat tomatoes in paprikash, Bolognese sauce, coq au vin, and one of my stalwarts, puttanesca sauce (see page 217).

Tom's method at that time called for removing the skins from the tomatoes midway through the roasting process, a painstaking operation. One day, the New Orleans chef (and a dear friend) Susan Spicer was visiting with us. When she saw Melinda laboring over the skins, she suggested that we blanch and peel the tomatoes before roasting. It turned out to be a lot less bother. Such adjustments are a vital part of the recipe process: there is often a way, revealed through long practice, to make a good recipe, like Tom's, better, or at least easier.

If we are serving the tomatoes freshly made or within a few days, I like to use garlic in this recipe. If frozen, garlic tastes old, so we discard the cooked garlic before freezing.

5 pounds plum tomatoes, firm but ripe (about 3 dozen)
2 tablespoons extra-virgin olive oil, or as needed
1 tablespoon coarse (turbinado) sugar
1 tablespoon *fleur de sel* (flaky salt)
6 to 8 sprigs fresh thyme
10 cloves garlic, unpeeled (optional)
Freshly ground black pepper

1. Preheat oven to 325 degrees.
2. Bring a large pot of water to a boil.

3. Line one large or two small sheet pans with parchment paper, and set aside.
4. Rinse and core tomatoes to a depth of about ½ inch.
5. Blanch tomatoes, ten at a time, in boiling water for 20 seconds. Transfer to cold water, peel, and cut in half lengthwise. Discard seeds, and place tomato halves, cut side down, on pans.
6. Drizzle generously with olive oil, scatter sugar, flaky salt, thyme, and garlic (optional) evenly over tomatoes. Add freshly ground black pepper.
7. Reduce oven to 225 degrees. Roast tomatoes until shriveled but still moist, 3 to 4 hours. Allow to cool. Discard thyme sprigs. Remove garlic skins.
8. If not serving immediately, discard garlic, top off with olive oil, and store tomatoes in one or two pint containers in freezer.

Sunday Frittata with Frizzled Leeks I began making frittatas regularly when our family transitioned from the pancakes-or-waffles-every-weekend phase into more "grown-up" breakfasts. As in much of my cooking, I believe I first learned to make a frittata from Julia Child, in one of her books or her television shows.

You can whip up a frittata for any meal: for a weekend breakfast, or with a green salad for lunch, or supper. The frizzled leeks are inspired by a dish served at Union Square Cafe in its early years. It was the first time I saw the word "frizzled."

"Fun word," I thought, and asked Danny Meyer where it came from. "My grandmother. Louise Meyer used to serve mashed potatoes with fried onions on top," he said. "When we opened Union Square Cafe in 1985, we substituted rutabaga for the potatoes, and leeks for the onions. That became our 'Mashed Turnips with Frizzled Leeks.' To avoid using the word 'fried,' I landed upon 'frizzled.' After that, frizzled leeks found their way onto everything from mashed potatoes to scallops, an omelet, red snapper, and just about everything except for ice cream."

If you don't have leeks, then thinly sliced onions, pan-roasted asparagus tips, crisped bacon all work fine. Concerning culinary substitution, I think of the Russian proverb that my grandpa Jan would trot out about many things in life: "If no fish, then lobster will do." Apparently, lobster prices under the czar were less steep than they are in present-day America, but I took his point.

As I noted earlier, Parmesan cheese has a lot of umami, which contributes to the high FPC of this recipe, especially when I top the finished frittata with some cherry tomatoes charred at high heat and pepped up with crushed red-pepper flakes.

SERVES 4

2 leeks, halved, cut lengthwise into strips no wider than a strand of spaghetti, and *very well rinsed* to remove all grit
3 tablespoons olive oil
8 to 10 eggs, lightly whisked
½ cup freshly grated Parmesan cheese
Freshly ground black pepper
Coarse salt to taste

1. Preheat oven to 350 degrees.
2. In an ovenproof skillet, sauté the leeks in 2 tablespoons olive oil over very low heat (just the hint of a sizzling sound) for about 10 to 15 minutes until crispy and golden brown.
3. Remove from skillet and set aside.
4. In the same ovenproof skillet, add remaining olive oil and heat for 30 seconds. Pour in whisked eggs.

5. Adjust heat to low (just above simmer), and let the eggs begin to set, undisturbed for a minute.
6. Remove skillet from stove, and place in the top third of the oven.
7. After 3 or 4 minutes, check to see how cooked the eggs are. They should still be slightly runny in the middle.
8. Taking a small handful at a time, distribute the leeks over the eggs and continue to cook.
9. After 2 more minutes, turn the oven to broil setting. Sprinkle the grated cheese over the entire surface of the eggs.
10. Broil for 1 to 2 minutes. The frittata will puff up, and the edges should be golden brown.
11. Season with black pepper and salt.
12. Cut into pielike wedges, and serve.

Pasta Pete-a-nesca My own variation on puttanesca sauce—hence the pun. If you have ever read a recipe for this, no doubt you have come across the tale that it was invented by Neapolitan prostitutes because it could be thrown together quickly. Like many food legends, this one is plausible but improbable. It takes me at least a half-hour to make, which would be a lot of wasted time if you are trying to move a stream of customers through a service business.

You'll note that I cook the tomatoes with the leftover rind of a Parmesan cheese. We never throw these out. When they are no longer grate-worthy, we freeze the rinds and use them in soups and stews and sauces. In this sauce they add extra umami to an already powerful combination of anchovies and tomatoes. Yeah, I know what "they"—the people who write Italian recipes—say about never adding cheese to a seafood sauce. Don't listen to them. It is the sheer force of all these flavors that makes this sauce ideal with whole-grain pastas. You won't miss the slitheriness of white pasta. I probably make this twenty times over the course of the winter and never tire of it.

SERVES 4

Salt to taste (for pasta water)
3 tablespoons olive oil
2 cloves garlic, diced
6 anchovy fillets (or more if you like)
2 tablespoons capers
½ cup pitted oil-cured black olives
¼ cup white wine, or juice of 1 lemon
2 cups oven-roasted tomatoes (see page 213), roughly chopped, or one 28-ounce can whole plum tomatoes with their liquid, roughly chopped
1 rind of Parmesan, pecorino, or other aged, hard Italian grating cheese
Crushed red-pepper flakes to taste
1 teaspoon sugar, or to taste (optional)
1 pound whole-grain pasta, such as penne, spaghetti, or linguine
½ cup chopped fresh parsley

1. Bring pasta water to boil, add salt, and lower to simmer.
2. Over medium-low heat, film a skillet with olive oil, add garlic and anchovies, and sauté, occasionally stirring and mashing anchovies until they dissolve and the garlic is golden.
3. Add capers and olives to skillet, and continue to sauté for 1 minute.
4. Add white wine, roasted or canned tomatoes, Parmesan rind, red-pepper flakes, and sugar. Raise heat to medium,

and cook, stirring as needed, until the sauce thickens, about 15 minutes.

5. While the sauce is cooking, return the pasta water to the boil, add pasta, and cook, stirring occasionally, until al dente. Drain pasta, reserving 1/2 cup water, and add this, along with pasta, to the skillet with the sauce. Add parsley. Toss pasta in the skillet to coat thoroughly. Transfer to serving bowl.

Farro and White Beans I was introduced to this recipe by Renzo Menesini, a professor at the University of Lucca, in Tuscany. In medieval times, Lucca was known as Europe's leading center for the study of herbal medicine. Renzo's academic specialty was painkilling herbs, which he researched each winter on extensive trips to Southeast Asia. He was a complete and courtly hedonist. I'll never forget the first time Melinda and I visited his home, a modern building unlike the rusticated and renovated farmhouses that newly arrived Tuscany lovers favor. On a towel bar in one bathroom of this consummate bachelor pad there hung some interesting black lingerie.

"My girlfriend's . . . ," the professor explained with a wistful smile.

Renzo once gave me a recipe with the most vivid headnote ever. It was for breast of chicken in a white sauce with pomegranate seeds. "Cover the breast with the white sauce and then add the pomegranate," he wrote. "The seeds will look like drops of blood on the white belly of an *odalisque.*"

Now, that's an introduction that gets your attention!

The following recipe, adapted from Renzo's *Le erbe aromatiche in cucina,* is traditional in Lucca.

SERVES 4

1 cup small white beans (navy, cannellini, Great Northern)
1 cup farro*
A few sprigs fresh thyme and parsley, tied in a bundle
3 tablespoons olive oil
1 medium onion, diced
1 medium carrot, diced
1 rib celery, diced
8 cups water
Salt to taste
Freshly ground white pepper to taste
½ cup freshly grated Parmesan cheese
Fragrant olive oil (preferably extra-virgin) to taste
4 sprigs fresh rosemary

*If you cannot find farro, you may substitute barley.

1. Soak the beans overnight in cold water (or cover with boiling water for 1 hour, then drain and rinse).
2. After the beans have soaked, rinse farro, place in a bowl, cover with boiling water, and set aside.
3. In a stockpot, sauté the vegetables in olive oil for about 5 minutes. Add herb bouquet.
4. Add the drained beans and water. Bring to simmer, and continue simmering for 30 minutes. Stir occasionally to keep beans from sticking.
5. Season with salt, and continue to simmer until the beans are soft (usually 30 to 60 minutes, depending on how dry and hard the beans are). Stir as needed.
6. Remove two ladles of beans and vegetables and set aside. Discard the herbs, and purée the rest in a blender or food processor.

7. Add the purée and the soaked farro, drained, to the stockpot, along with the reserved beans and vegetables. Simmer about 40 minutes, until the farro is tender. Stir as needed. Add water if the mixture gets too thick.
8. When ready to serve, adjust seasoning and stir in cheese.
9. Ladle into soup bowls. Drizzle with olive oil, and place one sprig of rosemary on top of soup in each bowl.

Two Juicy Golden-Brown Roast Chickens Nothing so inspires the affection of a chef as a roast chicken, a sentiment that lives in the same room in the heart as love for Mom. It's the yardstick by which food critics often measure a restaurant. If you buy the best free-range chicken and then cook it properly, it is simple to prepare, flavorful, and foolproof. Treat it carelessly, however, and it's nothing special.

A few years ago I was at the annual Burgundy winemakers' dinner known as La Paulée in the city of Beaune, where the greatest Burgundies are auctioned. The winemakers had invited Daniel Johnnes as their guest of honor, in appreciation of all he has done for Burgundy wine as a sommelier and an importer. His wife, Sally, like my wife, is a schoolteacher and couldn't take the time away from her class, so I got Sally's seat. Drew Nieporent, a Rabelaisian restaurateur and bon vivant, best known for Tribeca Grill, Corton, and Nobu (among others), completed our group.

The dinner was a down-home *grande bouffe,* as only the French can do it. Nearly six hundred people filled the huge banquet hall. We tasted fifty of the best wines on the planet. Whenever the increasingly tipsy chorus broke into the traditional La Paulée song, that was the cue for all to jump to their feet and join in with full voices and synchronized hand-clapping.

In between these outpourings of bonhomie, a half-dozen mustachioed musicians played hunting horns. To achieve the full effect, they faced away from the crowd, which meant that the bells of their horns and their backsides were pointed toward us. At the conclusion of each song, they bowed, still facing away from us. The effect was of a bunch of rowdy collegians mooning. Between the toot-tooting of the horns and this backassward salute, the music had the inescapable subtext of an extended fart joke. Such barnyard humor is typical of the earthiness of Burgundy, less so of aristocratic Bordeaux.

The wait staff navigated the crowded aisles bearing aloft huge trays full of food, dodging the high-spirited revelers. I watched in awe when it came time for the cheese course. Each waiter carried a large tray of cheese in one hand and, with the other, manipulated a fork and a spoon to cut individual servings. One-handed cheese service can be a challenge when a stationary cheese board is on the table in front of me. So, the ability to dip and pirouette amid a boisterous Burgundy-fueled throng struck me as a near miracle.

At around the fiftieth wine (rough guess), we pushed back from the table and walked to town.

"I need a roast chicken!" Drew declared.

I ignored him. Surely it was the wine talking.

"Me too," Daniel said. "Let's see if Ma Cuisine [a popular restaurant in the middle of Beaune] is open."

It was late, but they were still serving, and, rather than look like a spoilsport, I joined my friends for a golden-brown, succulent, milk-fed (Poulet de Bresse) roast chicken, and, it goes without saying, more wine. It was, in the words of the *Guide Michelin,* "worth a visit."

This particular variation is my adaptation of Thomas Keller's roast chicken from his excellent *Bouchon* cookbook.

TO BRINE THE CHICKENS

1 gallon water

1 cup kosher salt

½ cup honey

12 dried bay leaves

Juice of 2 lemons

2 tablespoons black peppercorns

2 chickens, about 3 pounds each

1. In a 2-quart saucepan, combine 4 cups water with the salt, honey, bay leaves, lemon juice, and peppercorns. Bring to a boil, lower heat, and stir to dissolve the salt completely.
2. Transfer the brine to a pot big enough to hold two chickens plus the gallon of liquid.
3. Add tap water to make a gallon of water. The cool water will bring down the temperature of the warm brine, so you can start brining immediately.
4. Remove chickens from refrigerator, rinse, and place in pot with brine. The refrigerated chicken will further chill the brine.
5. Refrigerate for 6 hours, or overnight.

ROASTING THE CHICKEN

2 brined chickens (see above)

Canola or grapeseed oil to film pan

1 tablespoon fresh thyme leaves

1 cup chicken stock

½ cup red wine

1. Preheat the oven to 475 degrees. If you have it, use convection to distribute heat more evenly.
2. Remove chickens from brine, pat dry with paper towels, and let stand at room temperature for 20 minutes.

3. Truss the chicken. Using about 3 feet of kitchen twine, I crisscross the breast to pull in the wings, crisscross the legs a few times, and tighten. Finish with a simple knot.
4. Heat two 9-inch cast-iron skillets over medium-high heat. Film with oil. Season chickens with salt and pepper, and when the oil is hot, place one chicken in each skillet, breast side up.
5. Place the skillets in the oven with the legs facing the back, the hottest part, so the dark meat, which requires the longest cooking, gets the most heat.
6. Roast for 40 minutes. If there are hot spots in your oven and you notice some parts of the chicken getting too brown, rotate the skillets to even out the heat.
7. Check internal temperature: insert an instant-read thermometer between the drumstick and the thigh. When the thermometer reads 165 degrees (about 55 minutes), remove the chickens from the skillets and leave to rest on a carving board for 10 minutes.
8. Add thyme leaves to skillets, and baste the chickens with pan juices and thyme.
9. Add ½ cup chicken stock to each skillet, and, over high heat, scrape up the browned bits from the bottom of the pans. Combine the liquids in one skillet.
10. Add wine to skillet juices. Cook for a few minutes over high heat to evaporate the alcohol.
11. Cut chicken into serving pieces. Reduce the liquid by half, and serve over chicken.

A Foolproof and Dramatic Big Roast Fish If you ever want something different by way of holiday fare, this is a memorable change of pace from turkey, standing rib roast, crown roast of pork, and leg of lamb. I owe this recipe—and many others—to Francis Mallmann. About ten years ago, I was on a tour of the Argentine province of Mendoza with a bunch of wine writers. Francis, who has the top restaurant in the wine district, was asked to prepare a luncheon in the countryside for the Catena family, the country's most famous winemakers. The guest of honor was Eric Rothschild, of *the* Rothschilds, makers of Château Lafite.

We drove into the mountains and parked by a stream. Francis had stationed two of his chic wait staff by the stream. I don't know how one country got so many good-looking people, but that is one of Argentina's many charms. As we piled out of the car, the waiters reached into the bubbling and babbling brook and retrieved two bottles of white wine, which they uncorked, poured, and handed to us in real wineglasses: not the plastic or thick glass vessels that one would have expected in the outdoors. In case we developed a thirst on our stroll, more wait staff, recruited from the same handsome gene pool, were stationed along the way to keep our glasses filled.

Our destination was a chestnut grove where Francis had encased a whole salmon in a thick coating of salt and set it to roast in a makeshift outdoor oven. There was one level of wood fire below the fish, and one above. He calls this setup an *infiernillo,* which he translates as "little hell."

After roasting the fish for an hour, he recruited three helpers to assist him in removing it from the heat. He broke the salt crust with a mallet to reveal a moist, perfectly cooked salmon. He served it with a light sauce of lemon, oregano, lemon peel, and garlic.

Since that time, I have oven-roasted salt-crusted striped bass, bluefish, and weakfish. Every spring I cook a fifteen-pound striper for fellow anglers at the Orvis store in Manhattan. If you are feeding a big group, this is a great one-pot—or at least one-tray—meal, and as impressive as any roast.

If you are being religious about CI, skip the potatoes, but this might be a time to stretch the rules. Have one.

Note: don't worry about using so much salt. Because the fish still has its skin on—even its scales—the salt serves to seal in moisture and provide even heat. You may actually end up adding a little salt to your fish when you eat it.

SERVES 8

FOR THE FISH

8 medium carrots, scrubbed
Five 3-pound boxes kosher salt
8 cups water
One 8-pound striped bass, gutted but unscaled
6 medium Idaho potatoes, scrubbed
6 medium sweet potatoes, scrubbed

FOR THE SAUCE

2 cups olive oil
1 cup chopped fresh parsley
½ cup chopped garlic
½ cup fresh oregano leaves
Zest of 2 lemons, minced
Flaky sea salt to taste
Ground black pepper to taste

Combine the ingredients in a bowl and set aside.

ROASTING THE FISH AND VEGETABLES

1. Place carrots on a sheet of foil, and wrap tightly to make a sealed bundle.
2. Heat oven to 500 degrees.

3. Lay newspaper next to the sink, and place a sheet pan on top of the newspaper. There should be about a foot of paper on all sides of the sheet pan, to catch any salt overflow.
4. Pour a box of salt into the sink. Mix the salt and water by hand, about 4 cups salt at a time. It should have the consistency of wet spring snow. Add and moisten more salt as needed.
5. Fill the bottom of the sheet pan with salt mixture, and tamp down so that you have about an inch of compacted salt. Lay the fish on top of the salt.
6. Lay the foil-wrapped carrots on the salt, and surround the fish with potatoes and sweet potatoes. No foil is needed for the potatoes and sweet potatoes, since the skin protects their flesh while roasting.
7. Cover the fish and vegetables with more moist salt, as you would if you were covering someone at the beach in sand. Tamp the salt down firmly. It should cover the ingredients with a layer about 1 inch thick.
8. Very carefully place the sheet pan in the lower third of the oven. Depending on the size of the fish, you may need two people to do this. Bake until a meat thermometer reaches 150 degrees. Hint: I keep track of the temperature by sticking a meat thermometer (not instant-read) through the salt and into the fish, before I place the fish in the oven.
9. After approximately 55 minutes (this is an estimate; let the thermometer be your guide), remove the salt-covered fish and pan from the oven, and let rest for 20 minutes. You may need two people to remove a larger fish.
10. Tap the salt crust with a hammer or wooden mallet until it cracks. It will come off in big chunks. Use oven mitts or a dish towel to handle the hot salt. Discard the salt in the trash, or toss it into the sink and run water on it. Remove the

vegetables. With a pastry brush, remove remaining salt from the fish, and, using a thin-bladed knife, lift off and discard the fish skin.

11. To serve, use two large spoons to lift individual servings of fish from the backbone and transfer to plates. Place a carrot, half a potato, and half a sweet potato on each plate. Garnish with sauce and serve.

Pan-Roasted Fish with Lemon Wedges, Garlic, and Fennel One of my most interesting magazine assignments was a *Food & Wine* piece with Laurent Gras. At the time, he was the recently installed chef at the Waldorf-Astoria's restaurant, Peacock Alley. He had previously been the executive chef for Alain Ducasse in Paris (and, before that, at Ducasse's Louis XV in Monaco, both of them three-star Michelin restaurants). When Ducasse was planning the move to Paris, he deputized Gras and charged him with the task of coming up with a more northern, less Provençal menu. Ducasse suggested that his young chef go back to classic French cookbooks for inspiration, and with the help of a fat book-buying bankroll, Laurent collected first editions of the classic authors, such as Brillat-Savarin, Prosper Montagné, Jules Gouffé, and Henri Babinski (whose whimsical nom de plume was Ali-Bab).

Rather than cooking like the restaurant version of a cover band that does note-for-note re-creations of other people's hits, Laurent's method was to let the idea behind a recipe sink into his memory in the expectation that he could reinvent it after sufficient reflection. "I don't read cookbooks cover to cover, looking for recipes," he told me. "I like to browse for fifteen minutes, lay the book down, and come back to it later. I might begin with the idea of a stuffed vegetable from one book, a sauce for that vegetable from another, a fish to serve it with from another. The ideas stay in my memory. Then, when I want to create a menu, I sit down and I say, 'What do I really feel like eating?' It may take me a month to create a recipe. That whole time, it's like a constant conversation with these old chefs who still live in these books."

Laurent and I would meet from time to time and page through his books until we had enough new inspirations for the article. "Why don't I cook a few at your house?" he said.

A week later, he showed up with the ingredients for a beef tenderloin with olives and pistachios (a redacted Brillat-Savarin recipe that, as far as he was concerned, didn't need the black truffles from the original). Also, just for the heck of it, a whole foie (goose liver) that would have smoked us out of the house when he sautéed it if I didn't have an exhaust over my stove with enough power to suck up a Brittany spaniel.

And just because he had them, and they are so gastronomically non-PC, he brought a half-dozen ortolans—little French songbirds that were gorged on millet and figs until they were supersized. Traditionalists are said to kill the birds by drowning them in a snifter of Armagnac. Even to a heartless gourmet this feels excessive and brutal, which explains why serving ortolans is illegal, even in France.

The recipe was quite simple. Stick the ortolans in separate ramekins, and put them in a hot oven, where they confit in their own fat. To eat, you plop the whole bird, beak and bones included, into your mouth. Where other parents are keen to tell their picky children, "Shut up and eat your vegetables," I got to proclaim the line now immortalized in family lore: "Shut up and eat your ortolans." They were about the most delicious thing ever. Having done it once, though, I am out of the ortolan-eating business.

Of all the recipes that Laurent cooked for us that night, the following simple fish recipe is the one I continue to make, and it is always glowingly received. I have prepared it with cod, redfish, weakfish, and striped bass.

SERVES 4

4 tablespoons extra-virgin olive oil, or more as needed
1 ½ pounds fillet of firm white-fleshed fish, such as cod, striped bass, halibut, or redfish, cut into 4-ounce portions 1 ½ to 2 inches thick
1 teaspoon fennel seeds
2 lemons, each cut into 8 pieces
8 cloves garlic, unpeeled
Flaky salt and black pepper to taste

1. Heat oven to 325 degrees.
2. Film ovenproof skillet with 3 tablespoons good olive oil.
3. Over medium-high heat, place fillets in skillet. If there is skin, put them skin side down.
4. Add fennel seeds, and then lemon wedges and garlic. Season fish with flaky salt and black pepper, and drizzle some olive oil on each piece. Cook for 1 minute.
5. Tip the pan, and spoon hot oil over the fish.
6. Place pan in top third of oven. Roast for 6 to 8 minutes, until fish just flakes but remains moist inside.
7. Remove from oven. Place fillets on plates, and place lemon wedges and garlic alongside (they will continue to add flavor to the pan juices, but you probably don't want to eat them). Spoon remaining pan liquid over fish, drizzle lightly with olive oil, and season to taste.

Double-Cut Rib Eye I don't foresee myself ever making Michel Richard's seventy-two-hour short-rib recipe that I mentioned earlier, if only because a complicated and expensive *sous-vide* rig is not practical for a home kitchen. However, I often make his amazing double-cut rib eye, also known as a *côte de boeuf,* and, in less Gallic circles, as a "cowboy cut."

I first ate it at an impromptu chefs' supper at Citronelle. The meal was a far cry from the inventive gastronomy for which Michel is famous. We sat down around ten-thirty. Thomas Keller had just concluded a meal celebrating his *Bouchon* book. Two blocks away, Jacques Pépin had been promoting his latest book at a dinner at the Four Seasons Hotel. In addition to Thomas, Jacques, and Gloria Pépin, some of D.C.'s chef fraternity arrived as service wound down at their restaurants: Fabio Trabocchi (maestro at the Ritz-Carlton), Eric Ziebold (a Keller alumnus who now had his own restaurant, CityZen, at the Mandarin Oriental Hotel), Robert Wiedmaier (of Marcel's and Brasserie Beck).

We settled in at the long wooden chef's table in the kitchen. Michel uncorked a Côte-Rotie, which we downed as we devoured three imposing steaks. Also French fries cooked in clarified butter (I would probably pass on those today), followed by an Époisses cheese that smelled like carnal sin made edible; for dessert, seedless grapes rolled in chocolate and dusted with cocoa powder.

We attacked our plates with the gusto of hungry laborers after a day's work. Lots of finger licking and bone sucking; also *de rigueur,* war stories about cooking and customers that food professionals trot out at such gatherings.

This cut of meat, when prepared this way, is the equal of the very best Argentine beef cooked over a wood fire. The thick salty crust is full of complex beefy flavor, and the tender, marbled meat is succulent and flavorful: a harmonious marriage of Maillard and umami. If you make this in your home kitchen, be advised: it's a smoky process, so a good ventilating hood or a nearby open window (or a "who cares?" attitude) is called for. I like to serve the steak with a side salad of watercress and radishes, and a big red wine. If you gnaw on the bone—which I strongly urge you to do—this recipe will easily serve six to eight.

According to gourmet grill chef (not an oxymoron) Adam Perry Lang, seasoning the meat before cooking, and rubbing with wet hands, allows the meat to ooze and create a "meat paste" that helps to form a quickly developed crust when it hits the heat.

SERVES 6 TO 8

2 to 2 1/2 pounds double-cut rib eye on the bone
1 tablespoon coarse salt
1 tablespoon black pepper
1/4 cup grapeseed or canola oil
1 tablespoon olive oil for serving
4 sprigs fresh rosemary for garnish
Flaky salt to taste

1. Preheat oven to 300 degrees.
2. Season meat with salt and pepper, wet hands, rub in seasoning, and let stand for 10 minutes, till the meat oozes a bit.
3. Heat half the grapeseed or canola oil over high heat in a heavy cast-iron skillet. The oil should be about 1/8 inch deep. Place meat in hot pan and brown for 2 or 3 minutes. Turn the meat and repeat. Also brown the sides. Should take about 10 minutes total. If the oil becomes too hot, adjust heat.
4. Transfer the meat to a roasting pan. Roast in oven for about 20 minutes, until an instant-read thermometer reaches an internal temperature of 115 degrees.
5. Remove steak from oven, place on cooling rack, and rest for 10 minutes.

6. Heat remaining grapeseed or canola oil in iron skillet, and recrisp the meat over high heat, about 1 minute each on top and bottom (no need to recrisp the sides).
7. Slice, drizzle with olive oil, season with salt, and garnish with the rosemary. Or serve with chimichurri (recipe follows).

Chimichurri In Argentine cuisine there aren't a lot of cooked sauces. I once mentioned to Francis Mallmann that, in all the years I had known him, and even though he had trained in the great kitchens of France and Italy, I had never seen a stockpot in any of his restaurants. He said I surely must have overlooked some. What he would not dispute is that Argentines, Uruguayans, Chileans, and Brazilians like their grilled meat finished with bracing sauces made from fresh ingredients. *Salsa criolla, pebre,* and mandarin oranges (added to the Brazilian pork-and-beans stew known as *feijoada*) are all used to focus and embolden the flavors of beef, lamb, pork, fish, and poultry. Of these sauces, I believe that the greatest is chimichurri.

A gaucho without his ingredients for chimichurri is like an American cowboy (or major-league baseball player) without a chaw of tobacco. The mix of sharp, tart, spicy, herbal tastes and the roundness of olive oil pumps up the flavor of already intense ingredients. Traditionally the gauchos make their chimichurri with dried herbs. Francis uses fresh herbs. His recipe gets my vote.

MAKES 2 CUPS

1 cup water
1 tablespoon coarse salt
1 head garlic, cloves separated and peeled

1 cup fresh flat-leaf parsley leaves

1 cup fresh oregano leaves

2 teaspoons crushed red-pepper flakes

¼ cup red-wine vinegar

½ cup extra-virgin olive oil

1. Prepare the saltwater solution (*salmuera* in Spanish): Bring the water to a boil in a small saucepan. Add the salt, and stir until the salt dissolves. Remove from the heat, and allow to cool.
2. Mince the garlic very fine, and place in a bowl. Mince the parsley and oregano, and add to the garlic with the pepper flakes. Whisk in the vinegar, and then the olive oil. Whisk in the *salmuera* and transfer to a jar with a tight lid. Keep in the refrigerator. Chimichurri is best prepared one or more days in advance, so that the flavors have a chance to blend. Serve with *côte de boeuf,* or any cooked beef.

Praising Braising

When Daniel Boulud and I wrote *Letters to a Young Chef,* it afforded Daniel the chance to reflect on the role of cooking in his life. He is acknowledged as a gastronomic master, comfortable in many styles, but if the affection that comes through in someone's speaking tone tells you anything, I would say that, of all the ways you can cook meat, Daniel's favorite is braising. His voice drops to a low, quiet register when he speaks of how a chef nurtures meat when he braises.

Daniel is far from alone in this sentiment. When I worked on a cookbook about Le Marche with Fabio Trabocchi, he waxed eloquent—and full of familial affection—on the subject of *il lesso,* a multi-meat, one-pot braised meal.

Long cooking of meat, particularly necessary with unglamorous chewy cuts, permeates a house with aromas that grow stronger and more appealing by the minute. To chefs, braising means hearth and home.

Here are two recipes representing two different expressions of braising: one is deep, layered, a flavor bomb; the other, much less complex, a chamber piece versus a symphony.

First, the wine-braised oxtail that Gray Kunz and I did for *The Elements of Taste.* The tail is among the ox's most worked muscles, followed by the cheeks—which also take well to braising. The umami in the beef, ham hock, wine, and tomatoes lends tremendous depth of flavor. I use white flour in this recipe in spite of the No White rule. The amount is negligible. If I am looking for one dish to ward off winter cold with a tidal wave of flavor—this is it. The bonus is that oxtail is a very cheap cut. The leftover sauce is great for risotto.

Wine-Braised Oxtail

SERVES 6

4 pounds oxtail
Kosher salt
Freshly ground white pepper
½ cup grapeseed or canola oil
1 ½ cups peeled and roughly diced celery root
2 cups peeled and roughly diced carrots
2 medium leeks, thoroughly rinsed, thinly sliced
1 large onion, peeled and roughly sliced
4 cloves garlic, peeled

1 bunch fresh thyme

½ bunch fresh rosemary

3 whole cloves

2 bay leaves (fresh or dried)

8 to 10 white peppercorns

1 tablespoon tomato paste, or 4 oven-roasted tomatoes (see page 213), chopped

2 teaspoons all-purpose flour

2 bottles dry red wine

1 ham hock

1. Preheat the oven to 325 degrees.
2. Season the oxtail with salt and pepper. Heat the oil in a large Dutch oven or braising pan over medium-high heat. Add the oxtail and brown on all sides, about 10 minutes total. Remove and set aside.
3. Add the celery root, carrots, leeks, onion, garlic, thyme, rosemary, cloves, bay leaves, and peppercorns, and cook, stirring occasionally, until the vegetables are tender and browned.
4. Add the tomato paste. Mix well, then add the flour and mix again. Deglaze with red wine, scraping any bits sticking to the pan.
5. Return the oxtail pieces to the pan, and add the ham hock. Bring to a simmer, cover, and braise in the oven until the oxtail is very tender, about 3 hours.
6. Remove the oxtail and ham hock from the braising liquid. Set the oxtail aside. Take all the meat off ham hock. Discard the bone, and julienne the meat.
7. Strain the braising liquid through a fine sieve into a bowl, pushing the vegetables through the sieve to give body to the liquid.

8. Return the braising liquid to the pot, and bring to a boil. Reduce by one-third over high heat. Degrease and season with salt and pepper.
9. Gently rewarm the oxtail and ham hock in the braising liquid.
10. Serve over polenta, farro, or whole-grain couscous.

Dorothy Hamilton's White Veal Braise This braise is quite different from the brawny flavors of Gray's oxtail. Often a braised one-pot meal is a fusillade of flavor. This veal stew, simple and clear in its appearance and its flavor, is also a one-pot braise, only less aggressive.

Dorothy Hamilton is the founder of the French Culinary Institute, but, more to the point, she is a very good home cook with an easy stoveside manner. She made this simple braise for us on a very cold night (like minus five degrees) at her lake home in Connecticut. We stood in the kitchen drinking wine and chatting. Without our even noticing the passage of time, the stew appeared to make itself.

A light red wine—say, a Tempranillo or a Burgundy—is my choice with this dish, because the meat is so delicately flavored.

SERVES 4

FOR THE BRAISE

4 pieces veal shank about 2 inches thick
1 medium onion, peeled
2 ribs celery, cut in half
2 parsnips, cut in half
2 leeks, cut in half and thoroughly washed

1 carrot, scrubbed and cut in half
2 bay leaves
½ cup chopped fresh dill stems (reserve fronds for sauce)
1 tablespoon sugar
1 tablespoon white-wine vinegar
10 whole black peppercorns
Water to cover

TO FINISH THE SAUCE

3 tablespoons heavy cream
3 tablespoons white-wine vinegar
1 tablespoon butter
1 tablespoon white flour*
1 tablespoon salt
1 or 2 tablespoons sugar
White pepper to taste
Reserved fresh dill fronds

*I tried to make the roux with whole-wheat flour. It doesn't work.

1. Combine the braise ingredients in a large pot, and poach until tender—about an hour.
2. Whisk the cream and vinegar together, and set aside.
3. Make a white roux by melting 1 tablespoon butter, then mixing in the flour and cooking briefly, so that it thickens but doesn't brown. Swirl roux into the poaching liquid until it is all incorporated. If you feel it is too thin, you can double the flour and butter.
4. Whisk the cream and vinegar into the liquid.
5. Season with salt, sugar, and white pepper to taste.
6. Serve in wide soup plates. Garnish with dill fronds.

A Fresh Green Salad for Winter: Shaved Brussels Sprouts I had long ago resigned myself to the fact that the words "fresh," "local," "green," "salad," and "winter" did not go together, for the simple reason that there is little that is fresh, local, green, and salad-worthy is to be had at that time of year.

Then I ordered this salad at Frankies Spuntino, a local restaurant owned by my friends Frank Castronovo and Frank Falcinelli, who hosted the grass-fed beef tasting that I wrote of earlier (see page 25).

Yes, even in winter you can get reasonably good warm-weather greens flown or trucked in from other parts of the country, but Brussels sprouts, usually more local, feel of the season. They are brawny in taste, in the way of a winter's cassoulet or braised short ribs. Because Brussels sprouts have a funky taste, quite strong and sharp, you'd expect that the salad dressing would call for equally powerful vinegar. It doesn't. Lemon juice lends this winter salad a light note. When local Brussels sprouts are no longer in the market, the California stuff is fine.

In *The Frankies Spuntino Kitchen Companion & Cooking Manual,* they use Castelrosso cheese, which may be difficult to find. If I don't feel like walking all the way down Court Street to Caputo's deli, I use feta from the corner grocery or supermarket.

2 pints Brussels sprouts, outer leaves removed, trimmed, and bottom removed
½ cup extra-virgin olive oil
¼ cup freshly squeezed lemon juice
Coarse salt to taste
White pepper to taste
1 cup roughly crumbled Castelrosso cheese (or feta)
Black pepper to taste

1. Using a sharp knife, a mandoline, or the grating attachment on a food processor, cut the Brussels sprouts as thinly as you can, and set aside.
2. In a large wooden salad bowl, whisk together the olive oil, lemon juice, salt, and white pepper. Add the Brussels sprouts and toss.
3. Transfer to serving-sized bowls, and top with crumbled cheese. Finish with black pepper.

Winter Vegetable Roast with Maple-Mustard Vinaigrette Why do I love roast winter vegetables? For starters, because they are fresh, local, and seasonal. Unlike summer produce, they keep for a long time without losing most of their flavor. They feel like winter food: hearty, substantial, rib-sticking. Francis Mallmann quick-roasts them at very high heat in a wood oven until they almost burn. A home oven doesn't put out that kind of thousand-degree heat, but when something as simple as slices of Delicata squash are coated with a little bit of olive oil, sprinkled with kosher or coarse sea salt, and then roasted, they come out of the oven chewy, nutty, sweet, and savory. Part caramelization, part umami, and part Maillard.

This dish is a slight adaptation of a recipe in Yotam Ottolenghi's *Plenty,* which I came across when I was asked to be a judge in Food52.com's "Tournament of Cookbooks." In case you don't know Yotam Ottolenghi's work—you'd never forget such a fun name—he is a London-based Israeli chef who writes a vegetarian column for the *Guardian.* He is not a vegetarian himself, which makes me trust his recipes even more. In other words, he is neither ideological nor moralistic about it: his only aim is food that tastes great.

Caramelized and well-seasoned winter vegetables are fine by

themselves, but the maple-mustard vinaigrette lifts the flavors enormously. We made this recipe for a New Year's Eve dinner, and afterward I received ooh-and-aah e-mails from people about "the best vegetables ever!"

For sure, the company, the wine, and the other food had something to do with the reviews. But, taking all that into consideration, tell me, honestly, how often are people moved to praise a parsnip?

A few years ago I would have said you need your own roast tomatoes (see page 213) for this recipe, but now I find that Desert Glory or similar deeply flavored cherry tomatoes, though they don't hold a candle to real summer tomatoes, are fine when caramelized.

SERVES 8

8 medium parsnips, peeled or scrubbed
8 medium carrots, peeled or scrubbed
4 medium red onions, peeled and quartered
2 heads garlic, halved
½ cup plus 4 tablespoons olive oil
8 sprigs fresh thyme
4 sprigs fresh rosemary
Salt and freshly ground black pepper to taste
40 cherry tomatoes, halved
4 tablespoons lemon juice
4 tablespoons capers, roughly chopped
1 tablespoon maple syrup
1 teaspoon Dijon mustard

1. Preheat oven to 350 degrees.
2. Peel parsnips and carrots; depending on size, cut lengthwise in half or quarters, about 4 inches long.

3. In a large bowl, toss parsnips, carrots, onions, and garlic with ½ cup olive oil, thyme, rosemary, salt, and pepper.
4. Spread vegetables on one large sheet pan or two smaller pans, and place in oven. Roast for about an hour, turning vegetables once or twice, to get a nice crust on both sides.
5. Meanwhile, heat large skillet, and film with 2 tablespoons olive oil. Add tomatoes, cut side down, and caramelize (no more than 10 minutes). Sauté in two batches. Remove to bowl, and set aside.
6. While the vegetables are cooking, whisk together remaining 2 tablespoons olive oil, lemon juice, capers, maple syrup, and mustard.
7. Place warm roasted root vegetables on serving platter, and pour dressing over the vegetables. Top with caramelized tomatoes.

Tomatoes and Corn ("The Fire Song") I'll close with the first recipe I ever dreamed up. After graduating from college, I lived for the better part of a year in Woodstock, New York. This was the time when The Band was at the height of their influence, when Bob Dylan was holed up in his mountain home, writing about the joys of simple country living (on a rock star's income), when Van Morrison would drive his little orange Volkswagen Beetle down to the swimming hole by the Millstream Motel every day and dive into the cool mountain stream with the rest of us.

I had my introduction to serious cooking at the "soon-to-open" (but somehow it never did) restaurant of Albert Grossman, who was Dylan's manager, also Janis Joplin's and Peter, Paul and Mary's. Every night we would cook for Albert and ten guests, testing recipes. My job was washing pots and chopping vegetables (two invaluable skills for anyone who wants to learn how to cook). The pay was two meals a day, plus three bucks an hour, which was enough to get by (with gas at thirty cents a gallon and cigarettes at thirty-five cents a pack).

At that time there was another, less iconic, but no less great musician in town: John Herald—Johnny to his friends. He was the cleanest flatpicker I ever heard. His tenor voice was pure and clear. He was briefly famous as the leader of the Greenbriar Boys, the first New York bluegrass group to gain recognition among Southern traditionalists.

Johnny was also renowned among his friends as a mushroom picker. The Catskills abound in wild mushrooms, but only a few people are experts at gathering them safely. I'll never forget checking out the contents of Johnny's bachelor refrigerator: six packages of Yodels and four bags of frozen wild mushrooms.

One afternoon in mid-August, when the first great tomatoes were ready to be picked in the garden and the local corn was sugar-sweet, John threw some in a pot and left them to cook while he went tramping through the woods to forage for chanterelles.

When he returned, his house was in flames, totaled. The music community threw a benefit for him that was far more intimate than, yet about as star-studded as, the Woodstock Festival. John presented a new composition, "The Fire Song," which started with the line "The tomatoes and corn were on the stove. . . ."

Although the story in the song ended sadly, I still found something optimistic in the words . . . and appetizing.

A few weeks later, Johnny threw a fish fry at his new (rented) house. He fried up fresh bluefish—which show up along the New York coastline when corn and tomatoes are at their peak. Inspired partly by his song and in equal measure by the bounty of August, I made up this recipe and brought it along as my contribution to the party.

To this day, in honor of John, I make this dish at least once a summer, dredging one side of my bluefish fillets in cornmeal and cooking them in a big black skillet that I put on my barbecue (thereby not filling up the house with the odor of fish, which can hang around for days). If there is no fresh bluefish to be had, then some shrimp sautéed in olive oil and garlic. It is also a fine dish with smoked spareribs or grilled chicken.

As with many of my subsequent spur-of-the-moment recipes, I made this one with crisped bacon. I often use bacon, almost as a seasoning, whenever I am stumped, especially with vegetables, or fish, or braised meat. Come to think of it, there are very few dishes that cannot be improved with a little bacon.

4 tablespoons butter
4 to 6 ears of sweet corn, freshly shucked, kernels cut from cob
6 slices bacon, crisped, and chopped
Freshly ground black pepper
2 large ripe beefsteak tomatoes, roughly chopped
½ cup roughly chopped fresh basil

1. Over medium heat, melt the butter in a 9-inch skillet.
2. Add corn, and sauté for 2 minutes.
3. Add bacon, black pepper, and tomatoes, and turn up the heat.
4. Cook 5 to 7 minutes, until the tomato liquid partially evaporates.
5. Transfer to a bowl, toss with basil, and serve.

Acknowledgments

First, my agent, friend, and taskmaster, Mark Reiter, who had the idea for this book and worked me over with slave-driving zeal until I seemed to know what I was doing. My other agent, Lisa Queen, who looked at many versions of the manuscript with fresh eyes and always encouraged me, even when I had my doubts. My wife, Melinda, who blue-penciled every draft and kept sharpening this book long after my brain had turned into a marshmallow. Lucy and Lily, for their love, their critiques, and coming back for seconds. The editor who believed in this project and who gave me such extensive, thoughtful, and helpful notes: thank you, Andrew Miller.

As ever, Marion Rosenfeld for her counsel and general good humor. Miranda Rake for her research help early on. Also Sonya Kharas. Donna Gelb for looking over the recipes. Chefs Zoe and Emma Feigenbaum and food expert Courtney Knapp for their comments. Culinary historian Andrew Smith for separating legend from history. A huge debt to Dr. Steven Tay for the medical wake-up call. All the chefs, food writers, home cooks, and experts mentioned in the pages of this book, who were generous with their time, their knowledge, and their meals.

And, finally, in the words of Paul McCartney, "I'd like to thank my mum and dad, without whom . . ."

Index

A NOTE ABOUT THE AUTHOR

Peter Kaminsky wrote "Underground Gourmet" for *New York* magazine for four years, and his "Outdoors" column appeared in the *New York Times* for twenty years. He is a longtime contributor to *Food & Wine,* and the former managing editor of *National Lampoon.* His books include *Pig Perfect: Encounters with Remarkable Swine, The Moon Pulled Up an Acre of Bass, The Elements of Taste* (with Gray Kunz), *Seven Fires* (with Francis Mallmann), *Celebrate!* (with Sheila Lukins), and *John Madden's Ultimate Tailgating.* He is a creator and executive producer of the Kennedy Center Mark Twain Prize for American Humor and the Library of Congress Gershwin Prize for Popular Song, on PBS.

A NOTE ON THE TYPE

The text of this book was set in Garamond No. 3. It is not a true copy of any of the designs of Claude Garamond (ca. 1480–1561), but an adaptation of his types. It probably owes as much to the designs of Jean Jannon. Jannon's matrices came into the possession of the Imprimerie Nationale, where they were thought to be by Garamond himself. This particular version is based on an adaptation by Morris Fuller Benton.

Composed by North Market Street Graphics, Lancaster, Pennsylvania

Printed and bound by RR Donnelley, Harrisonburg, Virginia

Designed by Maggie Hinders